What People Are Saying About the Newbody Workout

"Six years ago I was the queen of excuses when it came to exercise, but I really wanted to be fit. I overcame my excuses by working out with a friend—that was the starting point. The enjoyment I got out of the social aspects became bigger than my excuses. Seeing my body change was so motivating. My arms toned up (something I never had before) and I lost weight too (15 pounds and several clothing sizes in a year). My daily chores became easier—I felt more energized and limber, could lift without straining and could work longer and go further. I continued doing Newbody through my most recent healthy pregnancy, and the postural training helped me keep tight in the tummy and supported in my back so that I never struggled with back pain throughout my pregnancy. Even though I didn't always feel like going, I always felt better during and after Newbody—and still do!"

—Sara, 38

"I find it really works. I'm very energetic and I love how the low-impact exercise has got me working my body harder. Using weights has made a difference too, and I love all the new and interesting moves."

—Linda, 60

"I've battled weight issues, lack of self-respect, and a low self-esteem my whole life. Newbody helped me make great changes to my physical appearance, and it improved my mental capacities and emotional well-being. The program provided me with an opportunity to challenge myself and reach higher and accomplish more in the gym and out. I turned my life around completely and changed my mindset to a 'lifestyle change' rather than a 'quick fix.'"

—Michelle, 39

"I've lost over 20 pounds, and you can finally see my waist after 20 years. I feel better and am walking much straighter. People have remarked on all the changes I have made and that has been a real morale booster for me."

ie, 54

"I've been doing Newbody for a little over two years.... After a Newbody workout, I'm in a better mood, even on stressful days, and I sleep better at night."

—Cloe, 50

"I have a bulging disc in my back, and as long as I do my physiotherapy stretches and exercises regularly, I don't seem to have a flare-up. I also do Newbody. It has helped me to focus on my core strength and my posture to prevent injury and decrease incidents of back discomfort. The focus on the core helps me to keep better posture when I work all day at my desk job too—and that's also beneficial."

—Angela, 38

"For the first 16 years of my life, I suffered with asthma. In order to breathe more easily, I would round my back and sit forward on my hands. Consequently I developed a very rounded back. As I grew out of my asthma, I started running, playing squash, participating and teaching fitness classes ... in short, I became a cardio junkie. But while my cardiovascular abilities were great, my posture didn't change. I started Newbody and have found that the focus on posture has helped correct a lifetime challenge to stand tall and straight."

—Joan, 51

"I am a 58-year-old retired educator. I have been doing the Newbody workout for about four years ... I feel that a toned and healthy body defies age—most fit people look younger than their not-so-fit contemporaries!"

—Nana, 58

"My Newbody workouts still to this day leave me feeling exhilarated, balanced, challenged, and satisfied, all at the same time."

—Kim, 40

"I was introduced to the Newbody workout 18 years ago and immediately fell in love with the concept of alternating sculpting with aerobic endurance. I have been able to maintain my muscle tone and my lower heart rate as I age and the workout is so gentle on my joints. Newbody is unique and uplifting.... The best aspect is that I always feel as though I've accomplished something after completing the workout."

—Bobbie, 47

"Newbody has seen me through post-pregnancy, the slip-slide changes that started in my forties, and the aches and pain of daily life. Newbody keeps my brain sharp and makes me feel young and strong."

—Amanda, 46

"I did Newbody throughout my three pregnancies. Newbody was the class I came back to first postnatal. It has made me more aware of stabilization and core strength when I am doing day-to-day things such as picking up my kids, lugging groceries, and even riding my bike. It is the class that I believe is the perfect complement to everything we do at the gym and at home."

—Nicolle, 36

"As a mother of two boys, aged 5 and 3, I don't know what I would have done without Newbody, as it helped me get fit before I became pregnant, stay fit during my pregnancies, and be active and fit after my pregnancies. During pregnancy, weight gain and transformation of my body shape left me feeling the impact, particularly in my joints and pelvic floor as well as through increased fatigue when I participated in high-impact classes. Newbody was the perfect solution as it was a high-energy but low-impact total body workout that was easy on my joints. After I gave birth, Newbody helped me work on my power posture and kept me standing tall so I avoided the 'slouched shoulders' that many new moms develop."

—Susie, 36

PENGUIN CANADA

NEWBODY WORKOUT FOR WOMEN

MAUREEN (MO) HAGAN is a licensed physiotherapist. She started working as a part-time fitness instructor in 1984 at a GoodLife® in London, Ontario. Today, she is vice-president of operations in charge of group exercise and instruction training at GoodLife Fitness® Clubs. Maureen is the creator of Newbody, GoodLife Fitness®'s exclusive group fitness class, and is highly involved in the development of education and training in the industry. As director of education for Canadian Fitness Professionals (Can-Fit-Pro), she administers nine conference curriculums annually and one of the largest fitness-education events and certification programs in the world today.

In 2006, Mo was named IDEA Fitness Instructor of the Year (making her a favourite around the world); she was named IDEA International Program Director of the Year in 1998. She is a Can-Fit-Pro and ACE-certified fitness instructor, as well as an adidas three-stripe fitness athlete.

Mo is a well-respected and sought-after consultant and media spokesperson. She has been featured and quoted in many consumer publications, including *Canadian Living* and *More* magazine. She is the author of *GoodLife Fitness®: 6 Weeks to a New Body*.

ALSO BY MAUREEN HAGAN

GoodLife Fitness®: 6 Weeks to a New Body

NEWBODY WORKOUT FOR WOMEN

6 WEEKS TO A FIT AND FABULOUS NEW YOU

MAUREEN HAGAN

PENGUIN
CANADA

PENGUIN CANADA

Published by the Penguin Group

Penguin Group (Canada), 90 Eglinton Avenue East, Suite 700, Toronto, Ontario, Canada
M4P 2Y3 (a division of Pearson Canada Inc.)

Penguin Group (USA) Inc., 375 Hudson Street, New York, New York 10014, U.S.A.
Penguin Books Ltd, 80 Strand, London WC2R 0RL, England
Penguin Ireland, 25 St Stephen's Green, Dublin 2, Ireland (a division of Penguin Books Ltd)
Penguin Group (Australia), 250 Camberwell Road, Camberwell, Victoria 3124, Australia
(a division of Pearson Australia Group Pty Ltd)
Penguin Books India Pvt Ltd, 11 Community Centre, Panchsheel Park, New Delhi – 110 017, India
Penguin Group (NZ), 67 Apollo Drive, Rosedale, North Shore 0632, New Zealand (a division of
Pearson New Zealand Ltd)
Penguin Books (South Africa) (Pty) Ltd, 24 Sturdee Avenue, Rosebank,
Johannesburg 2196, South Africa

Penguin Books Ltd, Registered Offices: 80 Strand, London WC2R 0RL, England

First published 2010

1 2 3 4 5 6 7 8 9 10 (WEB)

Interior photos: Jim Hockings/Off Broadway Photography

Manufactured in Canada.

LIBRARY AND ARCHIVES CANADA CATALOGUING IN PUBLICATION

Hagan, Maureen
Newbody workout for women : 6 weeks to a fit and fabulous new you
/ Maureen Hagan.

Includes index.
ISBN 978-0-14-317020-4

1. Exercise for women. I. Title.

GV482.H35 2010 613.71082 C2009-906285-2

Visit the Penguin Group (Canada) website at **www.penguin.ca**

Special and corporate bulk purchase rates available; please see
www.penguin.ca/corporatesales or call 1-800-810-3104, ext. 477 or 474

In memory of my mother
She is no longer with me in this world
But she will always be my motivation and guiding light

Contents

Preface

My Newbody adventure started during a vacation in 1991. I was a full-time physiotherapist at University Hospital in London, Ontario, and I worked part-time as a fitness instructor at GoodLife Fitness®. I took a backpacking trip through the South Pacific, and while I was there, I visited many health clubs in an effort to maintain my fitness regimen. I kept seeing—and participating in—a low-impact group workout called Newbody. Offered at all the popular fitness clubs in New Zealand and Australia, the class stood out as a completely new and different group exercise class. At the time, step and high-impact aerobics were all the rage, and both were typically highly choreographed and often quite difficult for the beginner to follow. Newbody, however, was a low-impact workout that used light hand-held weights along with easy-to-follow choreography. These classes were packed with people, and it did not seem to matter what your level of fitness was, as everyone was able to keep up—yet I found that I was challenged by the muscle conditioning and aerobic-based exercises. As a physiotherapist, I was impressed with the Newbody concept. I understood the value of weight-bearing, endurance-based strength training, as it helps almost everyone improve their posture and strengthen their abdominals and back in a way that they just would not get from traditional strength training.

By the end of my trip, I was hooked on Newbody. Back in Canada, I started to introduce my class participants to aspects of this easy-to-follow yet challenging training format, and they loved the exercises and were amazed at how this new form of functional training improved their cardio fitness, muscle strength, and definition. I began to experiment with the program's exercise techniques and developed the seven unique training methods that today make up the Newbody program at GoodLife®.

Soon after my return from travelling I was offered a full-time position at GoodLife Fitness®, which I accepted. Shortly thereafter, I met an extraordinary fitness instructor from Australia, Lexie

Williams, who had in fact created the original Newbody concept. Lexie and I became great friends, and she has been an amazing mentor for me over the years.

Little did I know when I started attending those Newbody classes in New Zealand and Australia that the result would be an entirely new and exciting fitness program that can truly reshape your body and change your life! As I tell the thousands of participants that I present Newbody to every year, you have no way of knowing what new and exciting opportunities lie ahead as you embark on your own Newbody journey. What I can say from my experience is that it has been a fun, exciting, and most worthwhile trip for me, and I am confident it will be for you too. Join me and feel the thrill!

Introduction

Welcome to my Newbody program, an amazing 6-week fitness and healthy lifestyle plan for women—an easy, convenient, and fun way to change how you look and feel. Newbody combines aerobic exercise and strength training with sensible eating and lifestyle choices to guarantee the results you want. You'll get fit, improve your health, and look and be the best you can be no matter where you are on life's journey. The program has lots of variety and it works for everyone—whether you're a working or stay-at-home mom, student, empty-nester, 9-to-5er, or shift worker and whether you love exercise, wish you loved it, want to lose weight, need to be stronger, or just had a baby!

Here's what the Newbody program is all about:

- **NEWBODY EXERCISE.** This is the heart of the program and the foundation to improving and better managing your overall health and appearance. My unique 30-minute session combines the best exercises based on innovative training methods for women's bodies, for a head-to-toe, inside and out workout at home or at the gym 6 days a week with 1 day off. The total body workout integrates heart fitness with specific strength-training exercises targeting all the major muscles women need to exert to increase lean body tissue and caloric expenditure. It is time-efficient, fun, and appropriate for all levels of fitness. We use light, hand-held weights (1, 2, or 3 pounds) and high repetitions to make sure you work your muscles and body in the way you need to get long-term results.

- **NEWBODY EXTRA STRENGTH.** To change the shape of your body and feel healthier, you *must* strength train. Strength training is imperative because it builds lean body tissue (muscle) and strengthens your muscles, including your heart. It also improves your metabolism, which changes the way you will look, move, and feel. To ensure that you stay committed and to enhance the value of this program, I've created three 15-minute Newbody Extra Strength routines to include in your weekly workout that will strengthen the upper, lower, and core regions of your body effectively—areas that women need to pay more attention to. The Extra Strength routines are easy to follow yet challenging. We use light (1-, 2-, or 3-pound) weights, along with body weight, as resistance to build the right amount of strength required for improving your fitness and function. The light weights also guarantee that you won't get bulky muscles or injure yourself. The Newbody Extra Strength routines are included in the Newbody Workout Schedule (see page 44).

- **NEWBODY SENSIBLE EATING**. Newbody Eat Right is an integral part of the program because what we eat plays such an important role in how we look and how we feel—and how we feel about ourselves. My sensible, practical nutrition plan, based on healthy eating guidelines, is designed to give you ways to take control of food choices and portion sizes—and to help you manage cravings, moods, energy levels, and metabolism. Healthy eating is as important as moving your body, and taking small steps toward eating right every day will help you strike the perfect balance between the calories you eat and the calories you burn. As you get fit and lean, you will see your body composition and shape change. My Newbody Sensible Eating program will help you make healthy changes, achieve your ideal body weight and shape, and give you more energy every day. You won't need to count calories or to diet ever again.

- **NEWBODY TIPS.** I have included lots of personal tips, advice, and tools to help support your new healthy lifestyle and reach the goals you dream of! This information is based on my expertise and experience as a registered physiotherapist and long-time exercise leader and coach in the health and fitness industry.

All the tools and information that you'll need to change and improve your body and your life are in this book. Having worked with thousands of female clients and club members since 1983, I know just how important and effective the right kind of regular and consistent exercise is to a healthy body, mind, and spirit. And keeping physically active really can improve your day-to-day quality of life. For a commitment of just 30 minutes a day, you'll have more energy, you'll feel stronger physically and mentally, and—take a look in the mirror—you'll like what you see! As you strengthen and tone your body and feed it healthy foods, you'll stand taller, look and feel leaner, move your body more energetically, and have more confidence and an enhanced sense of identity! No wonder women who exercise and eat right like their bodies more and age better.

The Newbody program adheres to all the scientific evidence that shows that regular exercise and healthy eating can add years to your life—and life to your years! I probably don't have to tell you (your doctor and countless health organizations likely already have) that a lifestyle that includes regular exercise and a sensible diet may help prevent high blood pressure, heart disease, some types of cancer, type 2 diabetes, osteoporosis, and, of course, obesity and weight-related conditions that can lead to disease or early death.

I created the Newbody group fitness program for GoodLife Fitness® almost 20 years ago ... and have been perfecting it ever since. Besides being a total-body, low-impact workout that's simple to follow and suitable for all different levels of fitness, what's unique about Newbody today is the careful methodology I have developed and incorporated into the program over the years—methodology that is supported by ongoing research and studies on safe, intelligent, and effective exercise.

Here is a quick overview of what makes Newbody so special (you'll find more information about these training methods in Chapter 2: The Newbody Program):

1. **MADE FOR A WOMAN.** All Newbody exercises are created for a woman's body and alignment. The exercises target women's weakest areas, accommodate for narrower shoulders and wider hips, and, with light resistance and high repetition, maximize calorie burn.

2. **STEPS IT UP.** Health Canada and other health agencies and organizations recommend that for better health, everyone should increase the number of steps they take every day to 10,000. When you finish a half-hour Newbody class, you've achieved one-quarter of the daily recommendation

(2500 steps). What's really fantastic is that those 2500 steps are more than the average Canadian currently gets in an entire day and will burn about 250 extra calories!

3. **IMPROVES POSTURE.** The workout incorporates exercises that strengthen your postural muscles and protect the spine against the stress of sedentary living and poor posture. (Poor posture caused by ergonomics, weight problems, and so on is a common cause of back and neck pain, and statistics show that up to 80 percent of North Americans will suffer from back pain in their lifetime.)

4. **DEFIES AGING.** Staying strong helps keep you young and can even reverse the clock. Newbody's use of 1-, 2-, or 3-pound dumbbells focuses on strengthening muscles that women use and need every day. The workout is weight bearing in nature, so you have to move your body against gravity. And remember, rather than bulking up, you're toning and lengthening muscles for a stronger, healthier, and more beautiful body and helping prevent muscle and bone loss that comes with aging.

5. **INVOLVES MIND–BODY WORK.** Newbody's easy-to-follow routines integrate "brain fitness" techniques that support cognitive health. You will have to concentrate a bit as your coordination improves, but it's worth it as you'll benefit both physically and mentally.

6. **FOCUSES ON FUNCTION.** All the exercises are similar to moves we make in everyday life. We're not working upper and lower arm and shoulder muscles so they burst out of our sleeves ... we're working them so we stand tall, move with ease, and can lift groceries, babies, and briefcases. (Mind you, toned muscles look good too!)

7. **IMPROVES BALANCE.** Muscle conditioning is the foundation of good balance, which is especially crucial to well-being in later life. Newbody includes balance training, which transcends into vitality and confidence in everyday life at any age.

At the same time, my Newbody Program accommodates the lifestyle issues that women have to cope with today. Most women I know are short on time and long on taking care of everyone else's needs. The Newbody Workout Schedule is designed to fit into your day. You choose the best time to exercise for 30 minutes at home or at the gym. Keep in mind that research shows that good health generally begins with at least 200 minutes of accumulated physical activity a week. And making a commitment to follow the Newbody program (30 minutes minimum for 6 days a week) gets you off to a great start! Face it: life is not going to slow down to allow you time to get fit and healthy, so you need to create the lifestyle you want so that you can have it all.

Remember that this is a 6-week program for good reason. It actually takes your body and your mind between 21 and 45 days to change a habit. This will vary depending on the desired change, but you need to give yourself at least 1 month to rewire your mind to accommodate your new exercise habit. Women's bodies are somewhat resistant to exercise, so giving yourself 6 weeks is the safest bet!

At the same time, all the Newbody exercises make the most efficient and effective use of your time, effort, and energy. During each segment, Newbody engages as many of the major muscle groups as possible so that you're moving your body the way it needs to move to maximize calorie burn and achieve the greatest physical results in the minimal amount of time!

The next stop for you is Chapter 1: The New and Improved You. I've included a health checklist, as well as great tools that will set you up for success and, more importantly, help you stay committed. For example, you'll be asked to think about your DREAM goals (why you want to complete this program) and to write them down. I encourage you to follow these suggestions because they are proven to motivate people to start and stick with a fitness program. Only about 7 percent of the population actually write down their goals. *If you write down goals, you'll be 97 percent more likely to be successful in your program.* Follow the program completely, incorporate the tips as they fit your circumstances, and be ready to achieve the type of fitness makeover you never thought was possible!

All set? Are you ready to create your new body?

1

The New and Improved You

My mother always told me that as I learned to walk in my first year, I learned to run! I never sat still, and as I grew up, I loved nothing better than climbing trees and playing hide-and-seek, hopscotch, and double-dutch. My mother enrolled me and my twin sister in skating and swimming classes, and I took dance and gymnastics too. I did well at track and field (high jump, long jump, and relay teams), rode my bike everywhere, and played Red Rover with friends at school.

In my late teens, I discovered running as a great way to channel my high energy and manage my moods. I also discovered fitness classes as a source for fun and camaraderie. My mom always said that feeling good about yourself made you a happier person across the board—and she was right. I quickly realized that when I was active, I was happy and my self-confidence soared.

Today my life is anchored by scheduled fitness classes and enlivened by activities that I do because they are fun, such as ballroom dance lessons and weekend walks with my husband. Physical activity is a mainstay of my everyday life, just like eating, brushing my teeth, and going to work. As a registered physiotherapist, I have seen first-hand what a sedentary lifestyle can do, and I want no part of the many health risks associated with being inactive.

Here is what regular physical activity can do for you (and your commitment to Newbody puts you on this path!):

- **BUILDS ENERGY.** Regular exercise revs up your metabolism, helps reduce stress levels, and improves your sleep—which means you have more energy to do the things you love!

- **INCREASES YOUR BASAL METABOLIC RATE (BMR)**—*and* the number of calories you burn. Strength training (also called resistance training) increases the amount of lean muscle tissue on your body and therefore the amount of calories you'll burn even when your body is at rest. A higher BMR will help you lose weight and manage your weight throughout your life.

- **BUILDS LEAN MUSCLE,** which makes your body look leaner and toned. As you burn fat, you'll lose weight and enhance the overall shape of your body. Looking better naked and in your clothes will make you feel sexier, and stronger too.

- **INCREASES SELF-CONFIDENCE.** Research has shown that regular exercise is good for your body, mind, and spirit. Having more physical strength and stamina, and achieving a healthy body shape and size, gives you a better sense of confidence and self-efficacy.

- **REDUCES MENTAL SLUGGISHNESS.** As you build physical strength and stamina, you will sit and stand with a healthier posture (you need the strength to do that), be able to think more clearly and concentrate longer, and even manage your blood sugar levels better. All these changes will help you to feel happier, make better decisions, and stay alert longer in the day.

- **HELPS STABILIZE MOODS.** By helping to balance blood sugar levels and hormonal levels better (by increasing production of the good, "happy" hormones and slowing down the production of the bad, stress-producing hormones), exercise can even reduce symptoms of depression by as much as 50 percent! Regular exercise helps to improve feelings of energy and overall well-being, and in studies it has alleviated depression just as well as medical drugs.

- **REDUCES STRESS LEVELS.** Just 30 minutes of moderately intense aerobic exercise most days of the week will help you reduce anxiety and chronic production of stress-producing hormones that lead to weight gain, obesity, and mood and sleep disturbances. Strength training and mind–body exercises (stretching, yoga, Tai Chi, and so on) are also beneficial for managing symptoms associated with stress.

- **HELPS REDUCE FOOD AND HUNGER CRAVINGS.** Not only does exercise help to balance blood sugar levels and hormones that influence hunger, sugar cravings, and feelings of fullness, but it also helps to build willpower and self-control.

- **HELPS CONTROL WEIGHT.** A combination of aerobic exercise and strength training helps maintain a healthy metabolism (better than just one activity on its own or none at all) by increasing lean muscle mass, which helps you burn more calories at rest.

- **IMPROVES FLEXIBILITY.** As we get older, muscles and joints stiffen up more quickly and frequently. Regular exercise helps keep all the joints well lubed (oiled) and all the muscles, tendons, and ligaments strong and resilient.

- **IMPROVES BALANCE AND STABILITY, COORDINATION AND MOBILITY.** These are necessary components of fitness, and they help reduce loss of function, the risk of falling, and subsequent risk of injury.

- **MAY HELP CURB HOT FLASHES.** Regular exercise helps balance the functioning of the endocrine system (ovaries, adrenals, thyroid, and pituitary gland) that is responsible for regulating metabolism, energy, and hormone levels. (Exercise also reduces the risk for muscle weakness, chronic fatigue, weight gain, hair loss, and premenstrual and perimenopausal symptoms.) Aerobic exercise and strength training, as well as mind–body exercise such as yoga, Tai Chi, and breath work or meditation, all contribute.

- **ENHANCES BONE DENSITY.** Aerobic exercise and strength training both contribute to positive stress loads on bones, which respond by forming new bone (density) or remodelling the bone to be stronger. This reduces the risk of osteoporosis and may even halt bone loss associated with aging and menopause (loss of estrogen).

- **IMPROVES FUNCTION AND RELIEVES SYMPTOMS** among people with osteoarthritis and rheumatoid arthritis.

- **CONTRIBUTES TO A SENSE OF WELL-BEING** and an overall improvement in quality of life. As my mother said, when you look and feel good, you have a more positive outlook and improved self-esteem.

- **REDUCES RISK OF HEART DISEASE AND STROKE,** as well as heart disease risk factors including obesity, high blood pressure, high cholesterol, and coronary artery disease, when 30 to 60 minutes of aerobic exercise is accumulated most days of the week.

- **HELPS PROTECT AGAINST COLORECTAL, BREAST, AND UTERINE CANCERS.** Physical activity is also one of the best ways to prevent being overweight, which is a risk factor for cancers of the breast, esophagus, gallbladder, kidney, liver, pancreas, and the uterus.

- **HELPS STABILIZE BLOOD SUGAR AND IMPROVE INSULIN RESISTANCE** (a risk factor for type 2 diabetes).

- **EXTENDS YOUR LIFE.** People who exercise regularly have calmer dispositions, significantly increased life satisfaction, and longer life expectancies.

- **CONTRIBUTES TO ANTI-AGING** and improves muscle strength, flexibility, and function in young and old alike. Those who exercise are less likely to have disabling physical conditions resulting from stiff joints, poor posture, back pain, chronic injury, and life-threatening falls.

FITNESS FOR LIFE

Toddlers are a joy to watch ... and with all the running, jumping, twirling, climbing onto furniture, and dancing they do, they get all the exercise they need. If only we could all maintain that level of activity! Exercise is a wonderful way to celebrate life, enjoy our independence, and deal with whatever we have to deal with. It equips our bodies with the strength, stamina, and suppleness we need for living every day, and it prepares us for the future.

As a young adult, getting involved in fitness activities is a great way to meet people (and specifically to meet a partner). Be adventurous and try different forms of exercise or types of fitness classes and sports to find activities that you enjoy and will do consistently to shape a healthy lifestyle.

Once family and career become more important, regular exercise can help control weight and build muscle to keep your heart and body strong and in great shape—and it can help you feel in control of your busy life too! It also prepares the body for childbearing by ensuring a healthy hormone balance and metabolism. (The rule of thumb pre- and post-pregnancy is to maintain or modify your program, not to stop or start something new during this time.)

As hormone levels begin to shift during perimenopause, regular exercise can help decrease symptoms, including hot flashes, mood swings, achy joints, weight gain, insomnia, headaches and mental fogginess, irregular menstrual cycles, and increased anxiety, worry, and depression. Strength training specifically is a great way to help you maintain lean muscle mass, which keeps your metabolism fired up and helps prevent weight gain. It also helps shore up bone and insulin tolerance and lowers risk for illness and injury. Mind–body exercise—such as yoga, Pilates, and stretching—helps reduce stress, anxiety, depression, and hormonal fluctuations, and provides opportunities for self-reflection and meditation.

After menopause (around age 50), women start to lose muscle mass more rapidly—so strength training is even more important. This is also a time when women often gain weight and increase their waist circumference, which increases health risks—exercise helps there as well. Weight-bearing exercise and strength training will slow bone loss. Participating in weight-bearing, strength-based exercise will help improve your balance and the functioning of your neuromuscular system (the coordination and communication between your brain and your body), your eyes (vision), and inner ear. Regular aerobic activity is beneficial to the heart, bones, metabolism, and even the mind (it increases blood flow to the brain cells and may help reduce the risk of developing conditions such as dementia). It helps keep off extra pounds that increase the likelihood of developing diabetes, high cholesterol, and heart disease.

BEFORE STARTING THE NEWBODY PROGRAM

If you're under 35 and in good health, you probably don't need a doctor to give you the A-OK to start the Newbody program. But if you have been inactive for several years or have any chronic health conditions (including any of the following), you should most certainly check in with your doctor before starting: high blood pressure, heart problems, a family history of early stroke or heart attack deaths, frequent dizzy spells, extreme breathlessness after mild exertion, or muscle-, bone- or joint-related problems. If you have diabetes, asthma, or arthritis, I'm sure you'll get an enthusiastic thumbs-up with pointers for managing any symptoms while you're working on your new body!

If you can't measure it, you can't manage it

Measuring helps you manage ... and this applies to anything in your life. If you wish to improve or just understand how your effort or behaviour is working for you, then you have to measure it. There is power in tracking your health activities and keeping your eye on the scorecard. Research shows that women who monitor their progress are more successful at reaching their goals. Keeping score of your health indexes will also provide you with a way to measure yourself against recommended minimum standards, whether it is the healthy number of steps Health Canada suggests you should take a day or your blood pressure or cholesterol level according to the guidelines of the Canadian Heart and Stroke Foundation or the Canadian Diabetes Association. Knowing this information will increase your awareness and accountability as you improve your score, and will also increase your chances of staying on track.

Here are six of the easiest and most accurate methods to measure your progress and watch your health improve at the same time. I suggest that you record numbers at the start of the Newbody program, midway through, and then at the 6-week point.

Blood pressure

Blood pressure is the force that your blood exerts on vessels as it moves through your body. It goes up and down depending on what you're doing (sleeping, making dinner, or exercising) and how stressed you might be feeling (whether you're impatiently driving in rush hour traffic, talking to your mother, or reading a book). A normal blood pressure is about 120/80 millimetres of mercury (mmHg) or lower. The top number (systolic pressure) relates to the force of the blood leaving the heart. The bottom number (diastolic pressure) registers the pressure on the vessels as the heart relaxes between beats. High blood pressure (also called hypertension) exists when that blood pressure reading is chronically above 140/90 mmHg with little or no exertion. Hypertension is known as the "silent killer" because you can't feel it and there are no symptoms. But hypertension is a major risk factor for heart disease and stroke. Your doctor can take your blood pressure or you can monitor it yourself—blood pressure stations are available in most pharmacies and some health institutions. If your blood pressure is high, your doctor or health professional will talk to you about how to lower it through lifestyle (exercise, diet, quitting smoking, and stress management) and medication, if necessary.

Body mass index (BMI)

BMI is a universally accepted standard (a ratio of weight to height) for determining a healthy weight range for adults. A BMI measure of 18.5 up to 24.9 is considered healthy for both men and women. A low BMI (less than 18.5) puts you at higher risk for health problems, as does a high BMI (25 and over). If you want to know your BMI, go online and find any number of websites to calculate it (for example, www.calculateyourbodymassindex.com). What you should remember, though, is that BMI doesn't take into consideration how your body weight is dispersed: the amount of lean muscle and bone mass to fat weight. These are important parts of your weight and health. Gather all the information and put it together for a total picture of the weight that you look and feel your best at.

MEASURE TO MANAGE

Your BMI	Today (D/M/Y)	In 3 Weeks	In 6 Weeks
Height (in feet and inches)			
Weight (in pounds)			
Calculated BMI			

Waist circumference

Taking your waist body measurement is an easy measure of overall health. To manage excess body fat and reduce your risk of heart attack, heart disease and stroke, high cholesterol, blood pressure, and insulin resistance (type 2 diabetes), you need to keep your waistline measurement less than 35 inches. The men in your life should have a waistline of no greater than 40 inches. Use a tape measure or seamstress tape to measure your waist at the smallest part around.

MEASURE TO MANAGE

Waist	Today (D/M/Y)	In 3 Weeks	In 6 Weeks
Circumference (in inches)			

Waist–hip ratio

The waist–hip ratio (WHR) is a measure of trunk fatness. If you only want to choose one method to measure, this is the one I recommend. Research has shown it's one of the most accurate in identifying belly fat. (Belly fat is now regarded as an indication of your health status and risks.) Here's the formula:

- Measure your waist in inches at the smallest part.
- Measure your hips in inches at their widest.
- Divide the waist measurement by your hip measurement.

- Lower risk: WHR less than 0.8 for women; WHR less than 1.0 for men
- Higher risk: WHR greater than 0.8 for women; WHR greater than 1.0 for men

MEASURE TO MANAGE

Waist	Today (D/M/Y)	In 3 Weeks	In 6 Weeks
Waist (in inches)			
Hips (in inches)			
Calculated WHR			

NEWBODY TIP: To take proper measurements, remove any clothing, belts, or accessories from the area you're measuring. Stand facing a mirror with feet shoulder width apart and stomach relaxed. Wrap the measuring tape around the part you're measuring. Make sure the tape is parallel to the floor and is not twisted. Relax and take two normal breaths. After the second breath out, tighten the tape. The tape should fit comfortably snug without depressing the skin. Still breathing normally, take the reading on the tape.

Weight

Most people have a scale in the bathroom, so this is an easy way to keep track of how exercise is affecting your body. While my general recommendation is to chart your progress three times during the 6-week Newbody program, if one of your goals is to lose weight, then it's okay to weigh yourself once a week. Weekly weigh-ins help women stay focused. But there is one important thing to remember: body weight doesn't take the makeup of your body into account—by that I mean the proportions of fat, muscle, bone, connective tissue, and fluid. As you begin to exercise regularly and make healthier food choices, you will lose fat and gain muscle, and your body weight will fluctuate day by day as a result. Muscle weighs more than fat, so the numbers on the scale might not change as fast as you'd like (unless you have a lot of weight to lose or you substantially decrease your caloric intake at the same time). Pound for pound, muscle takes up 30 percent less space than fat. Also, unlike fat cells, which continue to expand as they grow, muscle tissue becomes denser, weighing up to three times as much as fat. In fact, the way your clothes fit will give you a faster and more accurate indication of your progress. That's why I always say: "Why weight? Think *shape*."

MEASURE TO MANAGE

(Measure weekly if you have 5 pounds or more weight to lose)

Weight	Today (D/M/Y)	Week 1	Week 2	Week 3	Week 4	Week 5	Week 6
Pounds							

See for yourself

Dress up in your favourite item of clothing or outfit—whether it's a slinky black dress or a pair of jeans—and look at yourself in a mirror. What parts do you wish to trim and tone up? Are there "jiggly bits" that you would prefer to live without? Take a picture of yourself, in that favourite clothing if you like, and post it prominently as your "before picture"—on your refrigerator door, the bathroom mirror, or on your desktop. You may not necessarily love what you see, but keep in mind that as you work through the Newbody program and make sensible eating changes over the next 6 weeks, you will look better, feel better, lose a clothing size or two, and like yourself better! A recent body image survey showed that working out boosts body confidence—and that's whether your shape changes or not. Just being physically active improves body image: 96 percent of women said exercise makes them like their body more.

Women's bodies: we come in all different shapes and sizes

Just as some women lose or gain weight faster than others, some women will respond to exercise more quickly than others. This is based on a whole bunch of factors, including genetics and your body type. An ectomorph, for example—think of Céline Dion—is naturally thin, with lanky arms and legs. Ectomorphs tend to have fast metabolisms and may find it tough to gain muscle. An endomorph is wider in the hips than in the shoulders—think of

Marilyn Monroe. This body type tends to have a slow metabolism and easily gains body fat as opposed to muscle. A mesomorph is naturally muscular and can build muscle quite quickly. Madonna is a good example.

While it's fun and interesting to think about what your body type is, don't get stuck on it. All body types will experience some changes within a couple of weeks of beginning the Newbody program—provided you stick with it. What you'll notice most is that your clothes will begin to fit differently, your energy will increase, and you'll sleep better, resulting in less fatigue. Also, your muscles will thank you a lot, which means they may be a bit sore for the first week or even two. But that's okay because they really are just grateful that you're using them.

The bottom line is that every body reacts a little differently to exercise and healthy eating ... but no matter what your body type, my program can help you get fit and firm to look your fabulous best.

To get started, find your healthy weight, learn about your metabolic rate (see Chapter 9: The Newbody Sensible Eating Plan), and learn how to exercise and eat sensibly. Remember that keeping a journal (use the Newbody Journal template on page 210) will help you discover your body type too!

ESTABLISH YOUR GOAL

DREAM the possible dream—your new body!

Before you start the Newbody program, it's important to identify your overall Newbody goal and to create a plan that will help you reach it. I have developed an easy method to help you set your Newbody goal: I call it DREAM, which is an acronym for Definite, Realistic, Evaluate, Actionable, and Meaningful! Let me explain.

- **D IS FOR DEFINITE**. Be definite when you create your goal. Ask yourself, "What will I have achieved when I reach my goal?" This question will project your mind forward to the day you get there. To do this, you'll have to set a date for when you wish to achieve your goal. Then write your definite goal in the present tense, as if you've already achieved it. Here are some examples of definite goals: *I have lost 10 pounds. I fit fabulously into my* *new red dress, which I will be wearing to my high school reunion. I have doubled my upper-body strength and now can lift my 20-pound cat with ease. I can now run 2 miles. My old blue jeans fit perfectly now.* You'll be amazed by how definite goals written this way trick your conscious brain into action. Being definite and having clear, specific goals will motivate you and help you stay the course.

- **R IS FOR REALISTIC.** Your goal must be realistic. You must be able to achieve the goal in the time you have to do it—in the case of the Newbody program, that's 6 weeks. So the goal *I have lost 10 pounds in 6 weeks* means that you will have to lose 1.6 pounds a week, which is entirely possible and a healthy number to strive for! If your goal is bigger (that is, you want to lose 25 pounds or drop from a size 14 to a size 8), then determine a more realistic goal for the first 6 weeks, then the second 6 weeks, and so on. Breaking down your big goal into smaller, manageable definite goals will prevent failure because the goals are more realistic and you will have a much better chance of succeeding. This is the part of goal-setting that most people struggle with—they set too big a goal and then get frustrated and quit.

- **E IS FOR EVALUATE.** It is important to evaluate your progress daily and weekly to keep your goal a priority in your day. Some of the ways you can do this include weighing yourself once a week, trying on your new red dress once a week, or measuring the number of steps you take every day. For this purpose, I have created a Newbody Journal (see page 210) to help you keep track of your daily progress. It's a simple and effective way to record the food you eat and the fitness you do every day. Recording your input (food) and output (exercise) is a powerful strategy for success. Writing down what you eat helps you make more conscious eating choices. Recording exercise is motivating because it's a ledger of your hard work and dedication. As you monitor your progress and see all the changes and improvements over the next 6 weeks, you'll see what a powerful motivational and educational tool it is ... and you'll start looking forward to the time every day that you sit down to record your progress. Mark my words.

- **A IS FOR ACTIONABLE.** It's important to create small actionable steps with an appropriate deadline. It takes 21 to 45 days to change a habit and rewire your mind. For change to occur, you need to practise your new behaviours consistently day after day. Having an appointed deadline is important for two reasons. First, when there isn't a deadline, there's no urgency to take action. Second, having a deadline also encourages you to create a plan. Knowing the deadline (6 weeks for the Newbody program), you can break down your goal into weekly and daily action steps. I have provided you with a Newbody Workout Schedule (see page 44), which will take care of most of this part of the goal-setting. What's most important is that you convert your goal to a 6-week target. Remember also to create your goal with start and end dates in mind. Write "start" and "finish" into the exact dates on your calendar to indicate when you will start and finish the Newbody program. It may seem trite, but this physical action makes everything real and makes you accountable, which is important to achieving success and being committed to what you want to change.

- **M IS FOR MEANINGFUL.** The goal must be beneficial and important in your life—and it is, if you feel emotional about it. Think about your goal and the benefits, and note what types of emotions rise in your body. If you get teary-eyed or feel chills of excitement or even a little fearful when you think about your goal, then it's very likely that it's a meaningful goal for you. For example, maybe you have wanted to lose 10 pounds ever since your last child was born 6 years ago—and now you're finally going to do it. Or maybe you've just had a conversation with your doctor, who has suggested that unless you start exercising and lose some weight, you may have to consider taking medication for high blood pressure and possibly type 2 diabetes—you want to tackle these health problems more than anything! Or maybe you want to participate in the 5K CIBC Run for the Cure (for breast cancer)—and thinking about that brings up all kinds of emotions. Write down all the emotions that go along with achieving your goal. Attach the emotion(s) directly to the goal. For example: *I have lost 10 pounds and am so proud to have achieved my pre-pregnancy weight from 6 years ago. I ran the 5K Run for the Cure with my 16-year-old daughter, and she was amazed that I could keep up. I am off all medications for my blood pressure and diabetes and I am so excited to have a clean bill of health. I stand taller and feel happier now that my lower-back pain is gone.* To make your goal truly meaningful and motivating, take a few minutes to reflect on your goal for the Newbody program and jot down as many emotions or feelings that surface in your mind as you project yourself forward 6 weeks and see yourself having achieved this goal and all the health benefits that go along with it. Live in that moment to help your brain process the feelings so that you can experience them long enough to capture the emotions around them.

Write it down

As I mentioned earlier, writing your goals down gives you something to look forward to as well as fall back on. You want something that will challenge you, but you also have to believe it is realistic for you to achieve. It is not how big the goal is that matters. It is the fact that you believe it's possible that counts.

Writing your goal down is an amazing and powerful means to achieve it. Less than 7 percent of the population writes their goals down. But those who do write them down are 97 percent more successful in the end!

Mapping out your action plan is important to completing it too. The Newbody Workout Schedule on page 44 in effect maps out your 6 weeks for you in an easy day-by-day format. I've designed the program to be progressive, allowing your mind and body to move forward at a comfortable pace, with lots of variety. This super-flexible workout schedule lets you exercise when the time is right for you.

If your dream goal is to lose 10 pounds and fit into your sexy red dress (a benefit!), start visualizing yourself as having achieved your goal. Close your eyes and see yourself wearing that beautiful dress, feel it, imagine yourself living your dream. When you make your goal meaningful and achievable, you're halfway there.

Making note of all the reasons *why* your DREAM goal is so important to you is helpful too. It makes the DREAM real and motivates you to stay the course. Check off (✔ mark) why this goal is important to you (you may check off as many benefits as you like).

- ☐ I've wanted to lose weight for years.
- ☐ I want to look more attractive—and meet someone special.
- ☐ I want to be strong so I can lift my kids without getting tired so fast.
- ☐ I want to keep up with my kids in the playground.
- ☐ I want to improve my heart health—my mother died of a heart attack.
- ☐ I am tired of being so down on myself for not exercising.
- ☐ I want to run a 5K/10K charity road race.
- ☐ I want to improve my health overall.
- ☐ I want to lower some specific health risks.
- ☐ I want to improve my body image—and be more confident.
- ☐ I want to improve my posture.
- ☐ I want to reduce back pain.
- ☐ I want to be a healthy weight.
- ☐ I want to sleep better.
- ☐ I want (other benefits) ______________________________.

CREATE AN ACTION PLAN

Now that you have determined your Newbody DREAM goal, it is time to take action and make it happen. Taking action begins with a commitment on your part to create a new mindset around fitness, food, your health, and your needs. You must also create an action plan for the program. An action plan will help you stick with the program—and the first 6 weeks of starting an exercise program are crucial because this is when women are most likely to drop out. Why is that? Women say the main reasons they stop shy of achieving their goals are that they don't have enough free time, they lack discipline or confidence when exercising, and friends and family are unsupportive. We're going to tackle those obstacles.

Ready, set, go!

Here are some proven and effective ways to help you make the Newbody program a part of your everyday life.

- **SCHEDULING.** Everyone knows that finding time to exercise can be a challenge. To make it easier, schedule time to exercise as you would any other appointment. Don't worry about when fitness fits into your day (morning, noon, or night), just make it fit. Also, don't worry about doing it at the same time every day. On the days you're doing two 15-minute Newbody Extra Strength routines, you can be flexible. If you're having a busy day, you can do these two 15-minute segments at different times of the day. Fit in one before you go to work, for example, and perhaps another at lunchtime or just before dinner. It really doesn't matter *when* you work out in your day—just that you do it! Do not let anyone cancel your appointment with fitness—not even you!

- **FINDING TIME IN YOUR DAY.** Think about the different ways you can make time for your Newbody workout. For example, if you tend to watch TV after dinner, commit to doing the Newbody workout for half an hour after dinner at least 3 days a week. Or commit to working through lunch so that you can leave the office earlier to get to the gym. Make working out a consistent part of your week—establish some form of consistency in scheduling so that you'll get into a positive behavioural pattern. For example, you could exercise Monday, Wednesday, and Friday at noon; Tuesday and Thursday right after work; and Saturday in the morning.

- **SEE YOUR SUCCESSFUL SELF.** Visualize your success as often as possible. Look at old photos of you when you were in your best shape. Imagine yourself doing the workout and feeling energized afterward. Get creative (with food preparation and planning) to ensure you eat less junk food and snack more healthily.

- **BE YOUR BEST COACH EVER.** Motivate yourself with positive language. Read inspirational novels or books that reinforce the message that life is not about how hard or long you work but what you do! Health and wellness is shaped by a positive attitude. Your body follows your mind, so set your conscious mind into positive motion with the words you say. Stand in front of your bathroom mirror every morning and tell yourself out loud, "I look forward to my workout and to eating healthily today." Be sure to meet yourself in the same mirror at the end of the day and honour yourself with a positive statement such as, "I did the best I could today, and that is good enough for me."

- **TRACK YOUR PROGRESS.** Keep an exercise and food journal to record your daily health-related activities (see the sample Newbody Journal at the end of this chapter and use the Newbody Journal template I've provided on page 210). This will motivate you to keep going and it will keep you honest. It will hold you accountable for every choice you make and will be helpful in reinforcing your good behaviours and establishing new and healthy habits.

- **STRATEGIZE.** Pack your gym bag the night before or put out your workout clothes and shoes for the next day so that you'll see them when you wake up. Make a date to work out with a buddy. Ask your family or friends for support, especially those who know your goal and wish to encourage you. At the very least, schedule your workouts ahead of time in your calendar. With these kinds of supportive strategies in place, there is a greater chance for success.

- **REWARD YOURSELF.** Besides your big 6-week goal, it's a great idea to give yourself something else to aim for in the meantime. Milestones and rewards are motivating. Here are some ideas for you to use:
  - **After 1 week,** reward yourself with a fun and useful fitness gadget, such as a step pedometer or heart-rate monitor.
  - **After 2 weeks,** buy yourself a great-looking workout bag or outfit.

- **After 3 weeks,** it's time for a night out with girlfriends.
- **After 4 weeks,** give yourself a pedicure.
- **After 5 weeks,** make a reservation at your favourite restaurant.
- **At the end of the program,** give yourself a new clothing item or treat yourself to a sleep-in.

NEWBODY TIP: Remember that the first 6 weeks of any new fitness regime are the most critical period for shaping new habits. It won't always be easy and you'll try to talk yourself out of doing it at times, but what I can promise you is this: it will be fun and rewarding. Be optimistic by staying focused on what you can do rather than on what you can't do. Focus on gaining rather than losing—gaining the health benefits that you checked off the list earlier in the chapter—versus what you have to lose or give up in the process. Being optimistic is self-empowering; it's taking back your self-control. The difference between those who succeed in life and those who don't is that those who succeed don't make excuses! They take action in the direction of their goals.

OVERCOMING OBSTACLES THAT SABOTAGE FITNESS

"I just don't have time"

This is probably the number-one reason many women never make it to the gym. Saying you can't get in shape because you don't have time to exercise is just an excuse for doing nothing. The way I look at it is this: fitness is all about health, and making time for your health will keep you in shape and give you more time to do all the things in life that you want to do. When you're in shape, you actually find extra time in your day. This is because you have more energy, make decisions faster, and have a higher tolerance for stress—which all adds up to give you more control over your life! Dig deeper to find the real reasons why you don't have time and seek to understand them—is it fear, fatigue, lack of knowledge, lack of self-confidence? Then strategize a solution.

"I want to, but ..."

"I don't have the energy/I'm tired," and "I don't have any discipline to stick with it" are the two most popular excuses for not exercising. If you tend to procrastinate this way, the way around it is to make fitness a part of your life one step at a time. There's never going to be a perfect time, a perfect day, or a perfect amount of energy to start getting active. And the universe will never gift you more time in your day. Review all the benefits or your reasons *why* starting a fitness program is important to you, and start by taking one small step at a time.

"I want results now!"

Change happens slowly, and it's unrealistic to expect your body to change overnight. As they say, "slow and steady wins the race." When your goals are realistic and planned with thought and strategy, you will be successful in the long run.

"I don't need a plan for fitness ... I'll just start"

You will need a plan, just like you need a road map to know how to get to where you want to go—otherwise, you will get lost. The Newbody program is a fabulous way to get started with fitness and enjoy all the benefits. It provides you with the guidance you need to do what you need to do.

"It hurts!"

Exercise will hurt once in a while, that's true. But it's good pain—and a sign that your muscles have been doing their job well and you have pushed yourself to get stronger. And please believe me when I say that all the benefits you feel (more energy, pride in how you're losing weight, changing your body, and improving the health of your heart) will more than outweigh those exercise-related aches and pains along the way. I often tell participants in my Newbody classes, "When your muscles hurt, they are really just thanking you for your commitment to good work."

"I hate fitness!"

This is where you have to flip the switch on your mindset. Cancel out "I hate fitness" and replace with "I like feeling more energetic," "I love my strong and pain-free back," and so on. Try to change your attitude and do the Newbody program with a positive and open mind. Making fitness fun (doing it with someone else, for example, or playing music you love while you exercise) is going to make the workout more enjoyable and go a long way in helping you to stick with it.

"Exercise is boring"

Not the Newbody program! The schedule changes weekly to keep you from getting bored. The exercises are designed to challenge and train your body and your mind in a way that is fun and far from boring. You will learn the moves and skills relatively quickly, and this will make you feel more confident and motivated to do more, and maybe experiment with other forms of fitness too.

Taking small steps and applying one or more of these strategies will not only change your body but will change you as a person—and you'll love all the changes!

SHOPPING CHECKLIST

- ☐ **SHOES.** For the Newbody program, you will need a good pair of fitness cross-trainers. This brand of workout shoe provides multidirectional support—for all the forward, backward, and lateral movements we make in the workout. Most cross-trainers have a wide outsole, which contributes to their stability. You also want cushioning at the heel and forefront for comfort and support. Mesh in the upper (rather than all leather) makes them breathable. The stability of these shoes makes them a great choice for Newbody Extra Strength routines as well.

- ☐ **CLOTHING.** Exercise clothing should provide a suitable fit and freedom of movement so that you're comfortable and self-assured. Cotton gets wet and stays wet, so I recommend

Q&A *with* Mo

Q **My friend just turned 40 and suddenly she works out regularly and looks amazing. She has lost weight and now looks more like she is 30. How did she motivate herself to do it?**

A First, you must decide if you're living the life you want. If you're discontented with your present situation, this will help you create purposeful change, which is a positive thing. By reframing that discontent as opportunity, you'll feel more energized (mentally and physically) and be ready to take action. Second, ask yourself, How motivated am I? You need to be motivated in order to be ready to change and succeed at it—only 20 percent of "potential changers" are ready for action, while the other 80 percent are still contemplating change. Understand that change is a complex and dynamic process that consists of six stages that range from "pre-contemplation" (not actively considering change), to "contemplation" (recognizing a problem and considering change), on to "action" (initiating change), then the "maintenance" stage (practising new skills and behaviours), and the last stage, where you complete the change process while fully aware that "relapse" (into old behaviours) can occur. Women may experience mid-life crisis as early as their 30s, which may explain your girlfriend's motivation and readiness to change. How ready are you? What is your motivation?

microfibre materials for function and fit. The newest microfibres are designed to transport moisture (sweat) to the surface of the fabric where it evaporates—so that makes you comfortable longer. Many of the moisture-management fabrics also resist odour and mildew. Look for soft, stretchy, and flexible tops with invisible or hidden seams for comfort (and less chafing). And moisture-management materials are just as important in the bottoms, whether you like hip-hugging shorts, baggy pants, or capris! It really is all about comfort, so get something that looks good and feels great. Some bottoms place the moisture-management panels where you really need the fabric to work: in the crotch, front, and back.

- ☐ **SPORTS BRA.** During exercise, a properly fitted sports bra is essential to comfort and performance. Look for sports bras that come in cup and band sizes rather than just small, medium, or large—they fit more precisely. Be sure seams and stitching are strategically placed for comfort. Anything that can chafe, will. Larger-breasted women might try a bra with moulded cups for firm support, while smaller-breasted women can wear a compression-style bra. But stay away from bras that look like cropped tops and provide little or no support. Wide, non-stretch straps or a wide Y-back panel increase support. High-performance breathable fabrics wick away sweat to minimize chafing. There are many styles of bras on the market, so don't shy away from asking for expert advice—especially when it comes to proper fit.

- ☐ **SOCKS.** Socks are a small but key aspect of comfort while you're working out. Breathability is important. For light activity, I recommend a breathable, cotton-blend sock or a high-performance sock that wicks moisture away from skin. Be sure to try socks on with your shoes. The right socks will make the most of the design features in your shoes. Good socks will keep your feet free of blisters too.

- ☐ **WATER BOTTLE.** I recommend reusable water containers such as Nalgene's Bisphenol-A (BPA)–free plastic bottles or one of the new stainless-steel containers.

- ☐ **TWO FREE WEIGHTS (1, 2, OR 3 POUNDS).** There are different kinds of free weights—I prefer neoprene or chrome. Either way, the 1-, 2-, and 3-pound weights are light. If you're a beginner, start with the 1-pound weights but buy a set if possible so you can work your way to a higher weight. Here's a guide:

- Iron and steel: The base for most dumbbells is iron or steel. These are the simplest and least expensive materials.
- Chrome-plated: The chrome-plating makes the weight look good. The coating may help prevent rust.
- Rubber-coated, neoprene, or covered with other cushioning materials: The covering helps protect weights against rust and floors against dings when weights get dropped. Neoprene contains latex, so if you're allergic, go with chrome or iron and steel.
- Other: Some rubber or neoprene weights are filled with sand or other materials. These weights are fine.

☐ **WORKOUT MAT.** Mats come in all shapes and sizes—what's most important is that the mat you buy is comfortable for your body. The mats used for stretching exercises or yoga are the type that coil and are made of a firmer and somewhat sticky rubber material. Any regular exercise mat with the proper thickness will do. When you buy your mat, be sure to unroll or unfold the mat onto the floor of the store first and test it out.

☐ **THE NEWBODY JOURNAL** is your conscience coach (to keep you committed and on track). Seeing your choices and actions on paper every day is an effective way to monitor your progress. It also keeps you honest and more accountable for reaching your DREAM goal. When you keep a journal, it naturally makes you reflect and spot trends in your behaviour (good, bad, and ugly) for better control and choices.

NEWBODY TIP: Wear a pedometer and step it up! A pedometer is an amazing gadget that clips onto your waistband halfway between your side and your belly button and counts the number of steps you take! Research has shown that counting the number of steps you do in a workout or a day is highly motivating. Participants of Newbody fitness classes are always amazed and overjoyed when they learn that doing the class adds about 2500 steps to their day, which is more than what the average person achieves in an entire day! For less than $30, which is the average cost, a pedometer is worth the investment 10 times over. You can buy one online and at most retail and fitness stores. Depending on how tech-savvy you are, choose a pedometer that's easy to use. Here are guidelines:

- **EASE OF USE.** At its most basic, a pedometers counts steps—if that's all you're interested in knowing, then look for a basic model. But if you'd also like to find out how far you've walked, how many calories you've burned, and other measurements, look at more advanced models.
- **READABILITY.** Look for a display monitor you can read in different types of lighting, especially if you'll be walking both indoors and outdoors.
- **CONVENIENCE.** A lightweight model should fit on the clothing you usually wear. Always try it on for size.
- **OVERALL STURDINESS.** Look for a sturdy clip and a security strap to hold the pedometer in place on your waistband.

Extras

☐ **MUSIC** that is fun, upbeat, and motivational will not only entertain you but will help you get better results. The right tunes allow you to exercise more vigorously and for longer. The rhythm and lyrics distract your mind from the work or the fatigue you may be feeling and also activate the same pleasure centre of your brain that food does. Choose a playlist (for your iPod or stereo) that contains songs with a rhythm or tempo that can be coordinated with your movements. There are many online music lists available to you to purchase and upload to your iPod or computer for your personal use.

☐ **FITNESS CLUB MEMBERSHIP.** Consider buying a membership to a fitness club for an energetic and supportive environment to work out in. You'll also have the opportunity to join in on group fitness classes or work with a personal trainer who can teach you how to exercise safely and effectively. Group classes are fun, offer instructional coaching, and add variety to your own program. Take advantage of the complimentary 1-week membership offer on page 215, with a value of $30—you have nothing to lose; give it a try!

SAMPLE NEWBODY JOURNAL

The Newbody Journal provides you with a daily checklist to help you record your workout and eating activities. I've provided a sample on the next page and you can find the Newbody Journal template on page 210. Use the template to make 6 copies (one a week) for your journal.

NEWBODY JOURNAL FOR THE WEEK OF: *January 2-8, 2010*

MY GOAL IS: *Start week 1 and commit to 6 workouts and follow the eating plan checklist*

	Monday	Tuesday	Wednesday	Thursday	Friday	Saturday	Sunday
Newbody 30 minute Workout	*30 min Newbody*		*30 min Newbody*		*30 min Newbody*		
2–15 minutes Extra Strength Training		*A & C Extra*		*B & C Extra*		*B & C Extra*	
Additional Physical Activity (minutes)	*10-min walk to and from office*	*10-min walk to and from office*	*10-min walk to and from office*	*10-min walk to and from office*	*10-min walk to and from office*	*30 minutes shovelling snow*	*20-min walk*
Total Physical Activity Time	*40 minutes*	*40 minutes*	*40 minutes*	*40 minutes*	*40 minutes*	*60 minutes*	*20 minutes*
Sensible Eating Checklist (✓)							
Breakfast	✓	✓	✓	✓	✓	✓	✓
Morning Snack	✓	✓		✓	✓		
Lunch	✓	✓	✓	✓	✓	✓	✓
Afternoon Snack	✓		✓		✓		✓
Dinner	✓	✓	✓	✓	✓	✓	✓
Optional Evening Snack		✓		✓	✓	✓	

NEWBODY DAILY EATING PLANNER

	Monday	Tuesday	Wednesday	Thursday	Friday	Saturday	Sunday
	Quick Nutritional Checklist (✓)						
4 Protein (meat/milk/alt) Servings	✓ ✓ ✓ ✓	✓ ✓ ✓ ✓	✓ ✓ ✓ ✓	✓ ✓ ✓ ✓	✓ ✓ ✓ ✓	✓ ✓ ✓ ✓	✓ ✓ ✓ ✓
3–4 Fruit Servings	✓ ✓ ✓	✓ ✓ ✓	✓ ✓ ✓	✓ ✓ ✓	✓ ✓ ✓	✓ ✓ ✓	✓ ✓ ✓
4–6 Veggie Servings	✓ ✓ ✓	✓ ✓ ✓	✓ ✓ ✓	✓ ✓ ✓	✓ ✓ ✓	✓ ✓ ✓	✓ ✓ ✓
5–6 Grain Servings	✓ ✓ ✓ ✓ ✓	✓ ✓ ✓ ✓ ✓	✓ ✓ ✓ ✓ ✓	✓ ✓ ✓ ✓ ✓	✓ ✓ ✓ ✓ ✓	✓ ✓ ✓ ✓ ✓	✓ ✓ ✓ ✓ ✓
8 Glasses of Water (circle)	1 2 3 4 5 (6) 7 8	1 2 3 4 5 (6) 7 8	1 2 3 4 5 6 (7) 8	1 2 3 4 5 6 (7) 8	1 2 3 4 5 6 7 (8)	1 2 3 4 (5) 6 7 8	1 2 3 4 (5) 6 7 8
1 Glass of Alcohol/Beer				*1 glass*	*1 glass*	*3 glasses*	*2 glasses*
I Feel Success (Yes/No):	*yes*	*yes*	*yes*	*yes*	*yes*	*Yes, need to drink water!*	*Yes, need more water, Mo!*

One thing I am proud of this week: *I completed all the workouts and ate more healthy foods (and meals too); more energy and having to write it down made me realize that I have to increase my veggies and limit how many glasses of wine I drink on weekends. Happy to learn that when I snack during the day, I tend to munch less at night (Uhm . . .).*

2

The Newbody Program

GET THE NEW BODY YOU WANT

I have trained thousands of women with the Newbody program for almost 20 years, and their success stories, featured throughout the book, confirm its effectiveness. They see their bodies change for the better and they live their lives more healthily. It is not just a fitness workout but a 6-week program designed to burn calories, build muscle, blast fat, and get you into shape pronto! To guarantee your success within 6 weeks, I have created a 30-minute Newbody workout combined with three 15-minute Newbody Extra Strength routines to be followed 6 days a week for 6 weeks in a row. My Newbody Workout Schedule (see page 44) shows you exactly what workout to do each day of the week. Each week is slightly different to ensure that you don't get bored mentally and do remain challenged physically as your fitness improves.

Each 30-minute workout will give you everything you need to increase your fitness level, improve your heart health, and strengthen and tone the muscles of your upper and lower body and core (abdominals and back). As your fitness level and physical body changes, you'll feel your energy, stamina, strength, and self-confidence increase, and you'll be able to perform daily activities with greater ease and enthusiasm. This is truly a unique fitness program!

NEWBODY'S SEVEN UNIQUE TRAINING PRINCIPLES

1. **NEWBODY IS MADE FOR A WOMAN.** All the exercises have been created with a woman's body in mind. I integrated female-friendly exercises, including:
   - Dynamic squats and lunges with a wider stance
   - Intentional weight-bearing exercises and sequences that mimic daily activities (such as leaning, lifting, twisting, and overhead lifting)
   - Upright abdominal and back (core) conditioning and integrated upper- and lower-body exercises
   - Resistance exercises that incorporate light, hand-held dumbbells (1, 2, or 3 pounds) to help women become confident with lifting weights

   Women's bodies are in general more resistant (stubborn) to exercise, so lifting lighter (1- to 3-pound) weights and performing higher repetitions is a safe and efficient way to achieve the results you desire, especially if you're just beginning an exercise program. The workout is low impact to help maintain and improve bone density without stressing the knee and hip joints or vertebrae (especially the lower back). This will not only help to preserve the strength and density of these weight-bearing bones and joints but will also increase the strength and endurance of the deeper stabilizing muscles around the hip, spine, and shoulder girdle. The combination of low impact and low weight with continuous movement and high repetition is what women need to get the results they want.

2. **NEWBODY STEPS UP DAILY ACTIVITY.** As I mentioned earlier, Health Canada and other health agencies and organizations, such as the World Health Organization, now recommend taking 10,000 steps a day for improving and maintaining health, maximizing cardiovascular health, and reducing the risk for lifestyle-related illness and disease. When you do a Newbody workout, you'll take a minimum of 2500 steps on average, or one-quarter of the daily recommended number of steps. This may not sound like a lot, but know this: those 2500

steps you achieve in 30 minutes amount to more than what the average Canadian currently gets in an entire 24-hour day! These steps add to your daily total as well as contributing to your fitness goal. The good news is that by adding 30 minutes of aerobic-based exercise to your day, you will almost double your number of steps and achieve almost half of your recommended daily quota of healthy steps. That's a great start.

NEWBODY TIP: As you increase your fitness and commitment to exercise, I encourage you to add an additional 500 steps a day until you reach your 10,000 steps in total. I also encourage you, especially if you're starting out, to track your steps with a step counter or pedometer. These are inexpensive and simple devices that you wear at your hip. They detect motion and track the number of steps you take. Just so you know, 10,000 steps a day through mainly walking is equivalent to approximately 5 miles, and 2000 to 3000 extra calories burned a week. Thirty minutes of more vigorous forms of aerobic-based exercise or activities—including power walking, low-impact aerobic fitness, step training, swimming, cycling, and jogging—will expend about 250 calories (depending on intensity or effort level) and accumulate 2500 steps minimum. It all adds up to good health.

3. **NEWBODY POWERS UP POSTURE** to improve the way you stand, sit, and move—and even sleep. Poor posture caused by prolonged sitting, poor sitting habits, excess body weight, and sedentary living is the most common cause of back and neck pain. Statistics show that up to 80 percent of North Americans will suffer from back pain sometime in their life. More than half of these incidents can be reduced to tolerable or zero levels when you're physically active—strengthening, stretching, and simply moving your body on a regular and consistent basis. Newbody teaches you how to power up and improve your posture by incorporating exercises that specifically engage the deeper core muscles (hip, abdominals, back, and shoulder girdle) responsible for maintaining normal posture (neutral alignment of the spine) in upright positions (sitting and standing). The exercises are also designed to protect the spine against excessive loads and stress that result from daily

patterns of movement, overuse, and excess bodyweight. When posture is correct, the spine is properly aligned from the crown of your head to your tailbone and the body will be able to perform efficiently and maintain its strength and suppleness. Newbody incorporates exercises and lots of coaching to help you strengthen your back and your body and change the way you stand, look, and eventually feel. Learn more about achieving a healthy back and how to power up your posture in Chapter 6.

4. **NEWBODY DEFIES THE NATURAL AGING PROCESS**. Exercise can slow the aging process, which is the breakdown of your body's tissues, including muscle, bone, brain, and heart. Staying strong helps keep you looking and feeling young and moving with ease and energy. For the most part, the Newbody exercises are designed to train your body to work against gravity by encouraging you to lift up and in opposition to the Earth's gravitational pull. This is very important, as it will help reduce stress and load on the weight-bearing joints. The type and amount of muscle work is greater, and the intensity higher—which means you will get stronger faster. Newbody uses light 1-, 2-, or 3-pound dumbbells and focuses on strengthening the "anti-gravity" muscles (back of the arms and shoulders, upper, mid, and lower back, gluteals, hamstrings, and calves), which women typically don't like to exercise. Why? These are usually the weaker muscles and you can't see them right away when you look in the mirror. Although you need those muscles to lift you out of bed or off the couch, climb the stairs, lift your child or carry the groceries, women would much prefer to perk up their pectoral (chest) muscles, flatten their tummies, and tone up their arms and legs. The good news is that you will be strengthening and toning all your favourite muscles as well as the ones that defy aging, which will power up your posture and help you move with ease, agility, and energy. And remember, you're not bulking up but rather shaping or toning for a sleeker, stronger, healthier, and more beautiful body. Strength-training exercise can actually rejuvenate muscle and make you stronger, no matter your age. The latest research suggests that strength training can turn back the clock on muscle aging at the cellular level. The actual struc-

ture of the muscle cell becomes impaired with aging but can be reversed and even take on a more youthful appearance. Remember, though: if you don't use it, you'll lose it. Strength training may be the new "fountain of youth."

5. **NEWBODY INTEGRATES MIND–BODY EXERCISES.** Newbody's easy-to-follow, intelligent sequencing of exercises uses "brain fitness" techniques that support cognitive health as well as other components of fitness involving the brain and the body—coordination, balance, and agility. Mind and body coordination techniques, including cross-body movement patterns, and the simple act of having to learn exercise sequences (otherwise known as "choreography"), are good exercises for your mind. Think about it. Your mind (brain) is just like a muscle and needs exercise and challenges too. Diseases whose incidence rises dramatically with age—such as Alzheimer's, dementia, Parkinson's aphasia, and even depression—all have their roots in mental health. Think of exercise as a physical crossword puzzle.

6. **NEWBODY MAKES REAL SENSE.** All the exercise moves we do in Newbody are similar to those we make in everyday life—in other words, we're not training to get bulky muscles but rather to have muscles for lifting groceries, babies, and briefcases. In fitness terminology, this is a training principle known as functional exercise. This principle also means that you won't waste your time performing one exercise or moving one body part at one time. All the exercises have a purpose—a real-life role to play—and are designed so that women will be properly equipped with the knowledge and exercises that prepare them for efficient daily living. The moves include striding/lunging, stepping and crossover stepping, leaping, intentional stepping, squatting, bending, sitting, leaning, lifting, and pushing and pulling in a wide variety of directions and against resistance. Newbody exercises will help women overcome natural weaknesses and instabilities more quickly than traditional strength-training machines. As a result, you'll increase fitness, body awareness, confidence, safety against injury, and performance in daily activities.

7. **NEWBODY KEEPS YOUR BODY IN BALANCE.** Achieving muscular strength, flexibility, and joint stability is the foundation of good balance, which is especially crucial to well-being later in life. There is a bit more to balance training than meets the eye. Here's what I mean (stand near a countertop or wall as you perform this balance test): Stand on one foot and find your balance. Now raise your arms in front of your body and overhead while following with your eyes. Repeat, lifting one arm out to the side and overhead while following with your eyes. How did you do? If you didn't lose your balance, try this. Close your eyes while standing on one foot. See how long you can maintain your balance. If you're like most 40-year-old or older women, you'll be surprised and perhaps shocked to discover that you can't hold your balance for even 5 seconds!

   Newbody contributes to better balance by incorporating exercises and sequences that require you to transfer weight quickly from one foot to the other, change direction quickly, and stand on one leg for prolonged periods of time while continuing to move your limbs—and that challenges your balance through the workout. Don't worry—I won't ask you to close your eyes; however, you should be able to do some of the exercises with your eyes closed and be able to maintain your balance. Often, I encourage my class participants to close their eyes during standing balance poses during BodyFlow or yoga classes. The ability to balance originates in the same area in the brain as motor skills. The brain translates information regarding the position of the body and coordinates the movement of our limbs. This requires coordination from many systems in the brain, as well as complex integration between skin, muscle, and joint receptors; the eyes for positioning; and the inner ear for head movement and position. Whew! It takes a lot to keep your body upright and balanced when you're standing or sitting, not to mention when you're moving.

   Even though balance is instinctive, you need to train it or else you will lose it, especially when your muscles get weak and tight, your posture changes, you gain or lose weight (including pre- and post-pregnancy), or even as your vision changes. You will, or perhaps you already do, notice yourself compensating.

You feel less steady on your feet when you get on your bike, step up on a ladder, or participate in more demanding activities such as skiing or skating. As a result you begin to slow down for fear of falling, and that is the start of a vicious downward cycle. You can, however, improve and maintain good balance throughout your life just by strength training. The Newbody workout integrates exercise and movement sequences that scientists and researchers use in their studies for testing patients. No wonder balance training has become one of the most popular components of fitness programs today.

Here's what Newbody can do for you:

- Increases muscular strength and endurance, and builds new muscle cells (not bulky muscles)
- Improves aerobic capacity and aerobic stamina and endurance
- Burns calories 24/7 and boosts your metabolism (or the amount of energy your body requires a day)
- Rebalances hormones
- Reverses insulin-resistance patterns
- Reduces stress levels and cortisol response associated with chronic stress and high levels of cortisol production by the adrenals
- Loses fat weight efficiently
- Tames mood swings
- Reduces symptoms associated with depression
- Increases circulatory levels of happy hormones in direct response to exercise (endorphins)
- Improves bone density
- Improves self-confidence
- Increases self-esteem (associated with changing body shape and strength gains)
- Decreases risk for falls
- Improves energy levels
- Increases quality and quantity of restful sleep
- Improves decision-making ability
- Decreases cravings for sugar and low-density carbohydrates
- Helps you make better nutritional choices

TIME, REPS, SETS, AND WEIGHT

When you exercise, you perform a certain move over and over for a designated number of repetitions (reps) to complete a set. When you perform one set or more of the same move without stopping for a rest, you accumulate time. If, as in the workouts provided in this book, a variety of moves are combined together in a sequence, it won't be necessary to take rest periods between sets because different muscles are working. This is one of many strategies for helping you see results quickly. The order of the exercises matters, especially when it comes to the Newbody Extra Strength routines. You will always start out with a simpler skill that involves the whole body, such as a squat with rear arm lift, a side lunge and lift, or a standing star sequence. Once the muscles are warmer and the mind–body connection has fired up, the focus of the workout goes from larger to smaller muscles and multiple joint to smaller, single-joint movements. For example, in the Extra Strength C core routine, you'll begin with a standing star sequence, move onto all fours (hands and knees) for an alternate arm and leg lift, move onto your belly for a back-strengthening exercise, and then move onto your back for abdominal training—with variations along the way. As you become fitter and familiar with the workout, the order of the exercises will not be as essential as it was in the beginning. In fact, it will be fun to mix it up, and your mind and body will enjoy the challenge of changing the order. Just reversing the order completely (floor to standing) will make the workout feel more challenging. Change is challenge.

I have predetermined how much weight you'll be lifting; when you first review the program, you might think that 1-, 2-, or 3-pound dumbbells is not a lot of weight. But take a closer look at the reps and sets. You will be performing more reps and sets than you would typically be doing in a traditional strength-training workout. The 30-minute Newbody workout is designed to be done on your feet. You are lifting weights and your body (it's a weight too) up and down, side to side, forward and back, and continuously performing moves that exercise the larger muscles of the lower body with the upper body simultaneously. This is going to be very different from performing a standing biceps curl, sitting triceps dip, or standing leg lift. The exercise effort or intensity will be further increased by the amount of weight you choose (up to 3 pounds), how you choose to progress the move (as shown), and the amount and length of rest breaks you take. You can measure your intensity, or rate of perceived exertion (RPE), using the simple scale below to measure your level of effort or work This is a basic tool to help you calculate how hard you are working, using the 1–10 as the measurement scale. The objective is to achieve a moderate (5–6) level of intensity within the first two weeks and sustain it throughout the workout. As your fitness and ability level increase, so should your intensity level (to 7–8). Depending on where you started you should be able to achieve and maintain at least 7–8 throughout the workout while occasionally pushing your effort toward a 9–10 on days you have the energy or motivation to challenge yourself in some of the exercises.

Review "Do It Right to Get It Right" (see page 40) to discover where you should start in terms of time, reps, sets, and weight.

0	Nothing at all
1	Very, very light
2	
3	Fairly light
4	
5	Moderate
6	
7	Somewhat hard
8	Hard
9	
10	Very hard

NEWBODY TIP: It's not how many repetitions you do, how many exercises you do, or how much weight you lift, but rather how you perform the move (with full range of motion, slow enough to control the movement with muscle) that makes all the difference. Think quality versus quantity and you will build a strong foundation for fitness. Consider also your starting level (see page 41) and learn your ABCs for executing the exercises correctly (see page 42).

BENEFIT FROM A PROPER WARM-UP

Warming up prior to exercise is an essential stage, helping your body transition from sedentary to active. It prepares your mind and your body for the upcoming activity. The warm-up is so named because the movements slowly increase your heart and respiratory rate and body's core temperature, which aids in warming up your muscles and tendons, lubricating the joints to increase tissue elasticity and joint mobility and reducing the risk of injury. The warm-up allows time for the heart to adjust to the increasing workload. The heart pumps more blood to the working muscles, carrying increased oxygen, nutrients, and hormones (glucose and adrenalin). The warm-up exercises mimic some of the exercises within the workout but at a lower intensity (without any weights or equipment). Think of it as a workout rehearsal. It typically takes 3 to 5 minutes to warm up, but as you age it may take longer (7 to 10 minutes). If you only have 30 minutes to work out, I recommend that you begin with 3 to 5 minutes, pick up your hand weights, and start into the workout at a lower intensity for one or two sets (5 minutes) to allow your body to gradually adapt and respond. Then give it your all for the next 15 to 17 minutes (leaving 3 to 5 minutes to stretch at the end).

TAKE TIME TO RECOVER AND STRETCH

I took stretching and flexibility for granted until I turned 40. But I have come to realize that stretching and flexibility are probably the most important contributors to preserving our posture and quality of life as we age. Just as you can protect your bones with strength training and protect your heart with aerobic activity, you can counterbalance the effects of aging by staying flexible. When you're flexible, you can move with ease, energy, and independence. Stretching reduces muscle tension and helps to restore the muscle to its original length. This helps to increase the resilience of our muscles, tendons, and supporting connective tissues. When muscles are flexible, they can more effectively support and stabilize the joints they surround to allow fluid and balanced movement of the body. The role of recovery in a workout is to stretch muscles back to their resting length after being put under tension, to alleviate soreness after the workout, to increase circulation within the muscle fibre, and to release tension in the body in general. The last 3 to 5 minutes of the 30-minute Newbody workout will focus on stretching to help maximize your flexibility and recovery from the workout. You will also learn how to stretch specific muscles within the three 15-minute Newbody Extra Strength routines.

Today many of the most popular fitness programs incorporate stretching to improve flexibility and restore energy balance after the workout or just a stressful day. Traditional mind–body practices such as yoga and Tai Chi are being integrated into fitness and cycling classes or offered as stand-alone classes. You don't even need to sweat to enjoy the benefits of these types of mind–body fitness programs.

Stretching is an integral part of any exercise program. Any Newbody stretches can be incorporated into your work, drive time, and recreational activities, and can be performed anywhere, anytime for so many good reasons. Stretching

- Improves posture
- Relieves stress—promotes relaxation in your muscles and your mind
- Increases circulation to the muscles; enhances blood flow and recovery, and reduces muscle stiffness and soreness following exercise
- Increases flexibility and suppleness of the muscles and tendons
- Increases range of motion at the joint, which influences posture and quality of movement and lowers risk of injury.

Stretch your way to a new body! Here's how:

- Stretch after your workout, not before, to reap the benefits of stretching when your muscles are warm and pliable.
- Hold each stretch for at least 15 seconds or 8 counts as follows: inhale "1 and 2 and"; exhale "3 and 4 and 5 and 6 and 7 and 8 and."
- Do not force the stretch beyond a comfortable point or bounce during the stretch. Stretching should be felt but not painful, and when you reach that "point of tension," hold and breathe. If you cannot do either, then back off.

- Breathe deeply and slowly using the in-breath as you begin the stretch and the out-breath as you release further into the stretch.

Always stretch both sides of the body with an option to repeat any stretches that feel tighter (muscles are shortened) on one side; for example, the front of your right thigh feels tighter than the left. This is normal, and stretching more on the tighter side will help restore muscle balance.

DO IT RIGHT TO GET IT RIGHT

The Newbody workout combines exercises into sequences that will help ensure that you maximize your effort (by recruiting the most amount of muscle) to achieve the desired results, faster. In almost all the exercises, you are moving your upper body at the same time as your legs while maintaining proper alignment at your core. This is a time-efficient and smart way to move—in that it mimics the way your body moves in everyday activities—however, you may find it a bit tricky at first. As you repeat the exercises 8 to 16 times, then repeat them again after another exercise as an exercise sequence, they will become easier to do and remember. The movements are meant to be performed with full range of motion and are continuous in nature (to recruit muscles and burn calories), but they shouldn't be performed fast. Each move should take an entire breath to complete. For example, as you squat down, inhale; as you lift up, exhale. As you step forward to lunge and your heel strikes the ground, exhale. As you lower into your lunge, inhale. As you rise up and return to the start, exhale.

Using your breath to pace your speed is a simple and practical way to control your speed of movement. I will coach you through every exercise in terms of when to breathe; lower and pull with your body; and exhale, lift, and press through the movement. To ensure you recruit as many muscles as possible in every exercise, remember to power up your posture: align your spine (stand tall or neutral), with your shoulders back and relaxed down (aligned directly under your ears), abdominals pulled in, chest lifted, and buttocks squeezed tight. This will guarantee you don't miss out on the best part of any exercise.

The Newbody workout's 15 essential exercises and 3 Extra Strength routines are illustrated by photos and a concise description: name, starting position, action, number of repetitions (reps) and sets, and progression (how you make the move itself more challenging, or how to combine it with the previous move or moves). Depending on your starting fitness and ability level, you will be guided on whether to use the 1-, 2-, or 3-pound dumbbells (hand weights). To make these workouts easy to follow, I have presented each exercise visually on its own and instruct you how to combine the exercises into a sequence.

If you have never worked out or trained with dumbbells before, that's okay: you'll find it very non-intimidating (the weights are quite light and easy to hold in your hands). You'll advance through a very quick learning curve, so don't get frustrated if it feels strange or too easy at first. Trust me: your muscles will appreciate you easing yourself into the workout. They will have not moved in quite this way before, and they will thank you for starting out easier, even though your mind thinks it can do more. Don't be surprised if you wake up the first morning or two after starting your Newbody workout with sore and stiff muscles. This is okay: in fact, it's great! It's all about getting your body moving again and your muscles "turned on." Celebrate the stiffness and muscle soreness with exercise. You may need to take a little longer to warm up your muscles and limber up those stiff joints.

The Newbody workout is designed to be continuous in nature. I encourage you to keep moving and not to take breaks between exercises. You may need to in the beginning, however, depending on your fitness and ability level, so consider your starting fitness level.

Just starting—go easy

Ease into the exercises. Start with fewer repetitions so that you perform the exercises more slowly. Progress your pace over the first 12 workouts (Weeks 1 and 2). As you become more confident and your body begins to respond positively, try to complete more repetitions until you reach the recommended number; then progress the number of sets as instructed. Start with 1-pound dumbbells (hand weights) for the 30-minute Newbody workout and the 2- or

3-pound weights for the Extra Strength routines. Once you achieve this, you're on your way and ready to take on more.

On your way—go harder

You are starting with some level of fitness so you should be able to complete both the recommended number of repetitions and sets for each exercise sequence as instructed, using 2-pound dumbbells for the 30-minute Newbody workout (3-pound dumbbells for the Extra Strength routines). Continue this for the first 12 workouts (Weeks 1 and 2). By Week 3, once you become more confident and your body adapts to the workload, you can progress the number of repetitions for each exercise as recommended. To ensure your safety, the intensity comes first, followed by the pace (or number of repetitions within the set amount of time).

Up and running—go for it

You consider yourself advanced and able to perform the exercises using 3-pound dumbbells to start. Complete the recommended number of sets for the first 12 workouts (Weeks 1 and 2), then increase the number of repetitions going into Week 3. Although you may be in good shape, you will need to give your body the chance to adapt to these exercise moves and sequences, as they are very different from traditional strength-training moves. It is safer and more effective to start at a slower pace, build your base level of fitness further, then go for it. You will understand once you give it a try. The total amount of work (when you complete the number of repetitions and sets) is surprisingly high and your muscles will feel the love!

EXERCISE EXECUTION—KNOW YOUR ABCs

- **A IS FOR ALIGNMENT.** Focus on proper alignment first. Set up each exercise with proper alignment (posture) to ensure that you're setting yourself up to target the desired muscles and body part and protecting your body against unnecessary stress. Execute the exercise movement with awareness of correct form and technique. This will become easier as you get to know the exercises and sequencing of them. Do not compromise correct form and technique for intensity or progression. Progressions are recommended only when you feel confident, typically starting Week 3 (following 12 workouts).

- **B IS FOR BREATHING.** Being aware of your breathing is important during exercise; breathing supplies your entire body with oxygen, and your breath helps set the pace and rhythm of your movement. In most exercises you should be breathing in as you perform the easy part of the move and exhaling on the harder part. To know if you're breathing correctly, listen to your breathing.

- **C IS FOR CONTROL.** Control the speed at which you execute the move. Your objective is to execute each move through its full range of motion. It is better to slow down your movement and move through a full range of motion than to move quickly trying to do more repetitions. Moving more slowly will give you time to focus on the desired action (as described for each exercise) and give it a "mental squeeze." Never compromise control or use momentum (swinging motion), especially when you're holding dumbbells. It may take you 3 to 6 workouts to learn how to coordinate the movement; get your mind into the move and your muscles firing and you will feel and see the difference.

THE NEWBODY WORKOUT SCHEDULE

Monday	Tuesday	Wednesday	Thursday	Friday	Saturday	Sunday
Week 1						
Newbody	Extra Strength A & C	Newbody	Extra Strength B & C	Newbody	Extra Strength B & C	Day Off
Week 2						
Newbody	Extra Strength A & C	Newbody	Extra Strength B & C	Newbody	Day Off	Extra Strength A & C
Week 3						
Extra Strength B & C	Newbody	Day Off	Newbody	Newbody	Extra Strength A & C	Extra Strength B & C
Week 4						
Newbody	Extra Strength A & C	Newbody	Extra Strength B & C	Newbody	Extra Strength A, B, & C	Day Off
Week 5						
Newbody	Extra Strength B & C	Newbody	Extra Strength A & C	Newbody	Day Off	Extra Strength A, B, & C
Week 6						
Newbody	Newbody	Extra Strength A & B	Newbody	Newbody	Extra Strength A, B, & C	Day Off

Day 7: a day off

The seventh day is a *free* day for you to do and eat whatever you like. Your body will be more forgiving than you think. As you increase your fitness and improve your metabolism, you'll be able to indulge 1 day a week. Can you handle it? Having freedom of choice (in what you eat and do) 1 day a week will allow your mind and body not to feel deprived or starved of the rest or foods you might otherwise crave. This will lower your chances of binging and you don't have to feel guilty for taking a day off. It's part of your Newbody Program. The emotions you'll feel after a couple of weeks will, in fact, be much different. You'll begin to feel that you no longer need those foods or want to be totally sedentary on this free day. (And don't be surprised if you feel lethargic or more tired on this day—that is your new body speaking, asking you to fuel it and move it more.) Soon you won't make unhealthy choices or sit around and do nothing. Your new body and new energy will crave the good stuff. So take the opportunity on the seventh day to make it a personal discovery day. If you choose to exercise on this day, choose something you enjoy—go skating, skiing, golfing, hiking, gardening, cycling, strolling on the beach, or window shopping. Enjoy your new body and new sense of freedom to be active and healthy! Schedule your free day on the day most convenient for you.

EXERCISE DURING PREGNANCY

Healthy pregnant women are encouraged to participate in aerobic and strength-conditioning exercise as part of a healthy lifestyle. Exercise post-pregnancy is especially important both for mom and for the baby. Quantity or quality of breast milk is not affected by exercise. Here are all the reasons why the Newbody program is ideal for pregnant women:

- Newbody is upright training—this means there is no concern of heart-rate changes with position changes or contra-indicated lying positions.
- The low-impact moves help strengthen the body while minimizing joint stresses.

- Functional strengthening exercises (upright abdominal and back-strengthening moves) help maintain and improve your posture and strengthen your lower back. Training in an upright position will help manage the weight of the baby on the woman's body during pregnancy and help restore core strength immediately after.
- Hip (pelvis) stability and strengthening support the pelvic floor (pre- and post-).
- Postural training strengthens and builds muscular endurance of the erector spinals. This helps to counter-support weight gain in front (breast and belly).
- Balance training is ideal for re-establishing balance with fluctuating weight gain and post-pregnancy weight loss.
- Newbody helps prevent excess weight gain before and healthy weight loss afterwards.
- Newbody helps manage hormonal fluctuations.
- Use of hand weights and specific upper-body strength training prepares new mothers for increased strength demands (carrying and nursing baby). And there's no worry about getting the heart rate up beyond the recommended levels with light weights. But of course, we still recommend that you monitor your intensity—see the next section.
- There are emotional benefits too. Participating in exercise provides a woman with a feeling of self-control and identity as her life changes.

Exercise intensity during pregnancy

Pregnant women should modify their exercise intensity while they are pregnant. Here are three ways to monitor your intensity to keep your heart rate within the recommended training zone for pregnancy.

1. **THE TALK TEST.** Exercise at a comfortable intensity so you can maintain a conversation during exercise. If you can't carry on a conversation, reduce the exercise intensity.

2. **PERCEIVED EXERTION** is a fast and easy way to monitor your intensity day to day and adjust accordingly depending on your

stage in pregnancy. Pregnant women should listen to their body and how they are feeling and aim to exercise between 5–8 on the RPE scale (on page 37).

3. **WEAR A HEART-RATE MONITOR** to measure heart rate during exercise and work within the recommended target zone determined by age:

MODIFIED HEART-RATE TARGET ZONES FOR AEROBIC EXERCISE IN PREGNANCY

Maternal Age	Heart-Rate Target Zone (beats/min)	Heart-Rate Target Zone (beats/10 sec)
Less than 20	140–155	23–26
20–29	135–150	22–25
30–39	130–145	21–24
40 or greater	125–140	20–23

Q&A *with* Mo

Q **What is the best time to work out? I've read that I will lose more weight if I exercise in the morning before I eat breakfast.**

A Whether you work out in the morning, at noon, or in the evening, the benefits are the same. If you exercise at a time that works for you, you will succeed at exercise and gain the benefits. This is one reason why I encourage you to keep a journal, so that you will learn what times work and don't work for you. What is most important is that exercise becomes a routine or habit that fits into your schedule well and that follows the FITT formula—frequency, intensity, time, and type.

FREQUENCY. You will exercise 6 times a week because this will create a healthy habit in your daily routine. One day off gives your body the opportunity to rest, rejuvenate, and reprogram for the next 6 days ahead.

INTENSITY. You will learn how to monitor your workout intensity and increase it as you get stronger, to achieve results.

TIME. The program is 30 minutes each day for 6 days, for a total of 180 minutes per week. That's the minimum amount of time required to achieve the numerous benefits associated with regular physical exercise and lower risk for illness and disease.

TYPE. The Newbody workout incorporates both aerobic and resistance-training exercise for an all-in-one workout, along with basic stretching (flexibility)—all essential for achieving your new body!

The 30-Minute Newbody Workout

15 ESSENTIAL EXERCISES

The Newbody workout is presented in this chapter in pictorial form to assist you in learning how to perform each exercise correctly along with an option and/or progression. Additional exercises will be introduced throughout Chapters 3 to 8 as complementary, bonus exercises.

At the very minimum, you will complete in a 30-minute Newbody workout:

- A 5–7 minute warm-up
- One aerobic sequence
- One functional strength sequence
- A 3- to 5-minute standing recovery (including active range of motion and flexibility)

The Warm-Up

It will take you about 5 to 7 minutes to complete the following 7 exercises, with each exercise being performed for a specific number of repetitions. Begin each exercise leading with your right foot, then repeat the entire exercise sequence leading with your left. This will integrate the mind and the muscles and ensure a balanced workout as well as give the body sufficient time to warm up.

MARCH WITH VARIATIONS: ON THE SPOT, FORWARD AND BACK, SIDE TO SIDE

Works buttocks (gluteals), quadriceps, hamstrings, abdominals, back, and shoulders

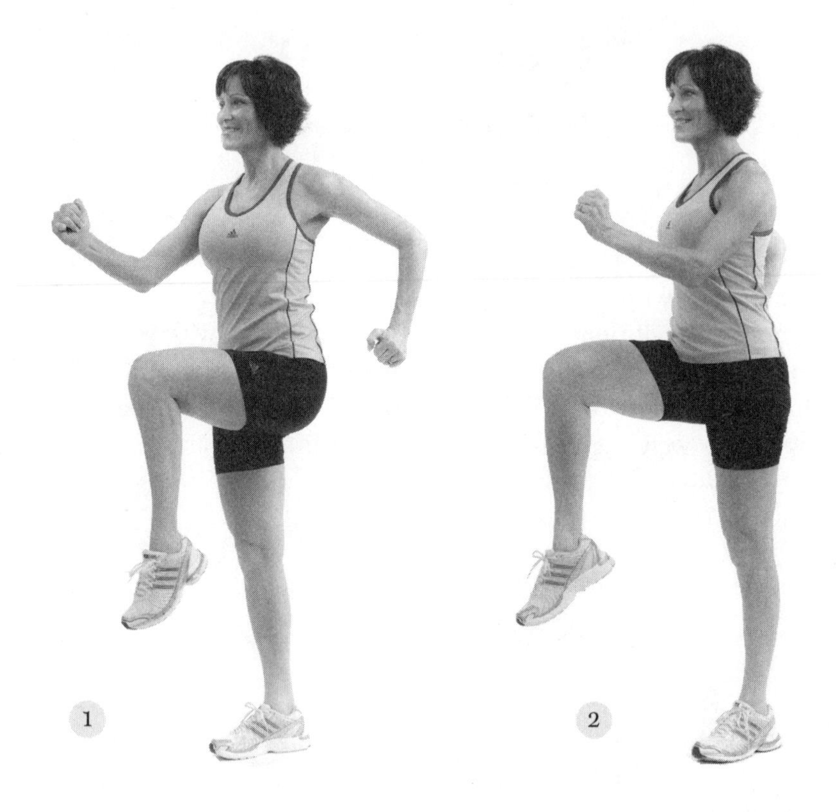

START: Stand tall (chest lifted, shoulders down, and abdominals pulled in) with feet hip width apart and arms at your sides with elbows bent.

ACTION: Lift knees high, in an alternating fashion, stepping on to the right, lifting left (1), then stepping onto the left, lifting right (2). This is 1 repetition. Swing arms forward and backward in a reciprocal action to the legs (1), (2); march in place as indicated.

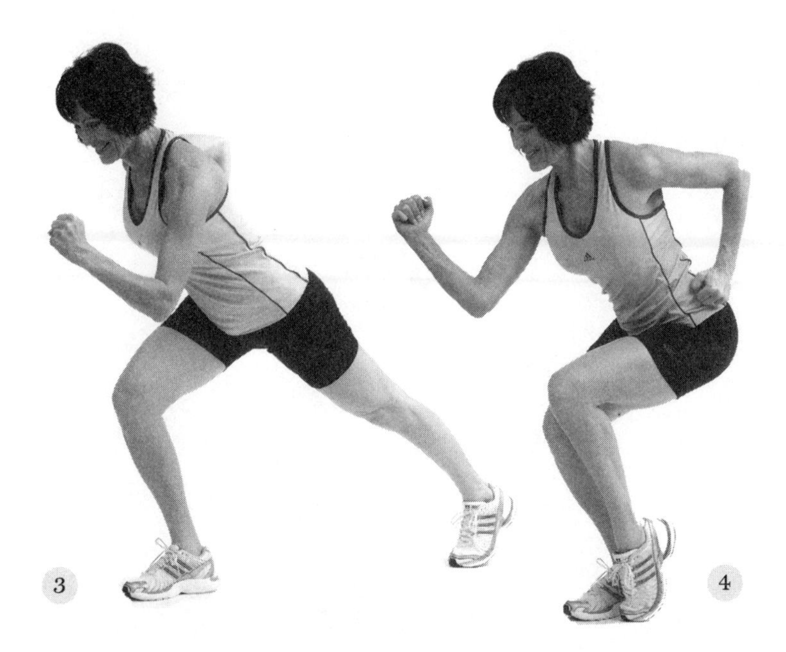

PROGRESSION: March forward and back (right then left equals 1 repetition) or sideways, crossing one foot in front or behind the other, then stand on your right foot and lean forward at the hips, reach your left leg back behind you to touch back, with heel lifted off the floor (3). Then pull the left foot in to touch alongside the right foot and pause (4); push back and repeat as indicated (repeater). Switch sides and repeat.

Repeat, starting on the right, 2 sets × 16 repetitions marching in place, 4 sets × 4 repetitions moving forward and backward, followed by 8 to 16 repeater moves on the right. Repeat the sequence starting on the left.

ALTERNATING FORWARD LUNGE

Works buttocks (gluteals), quadriceps, hamstrings, abdominals, and back muscles

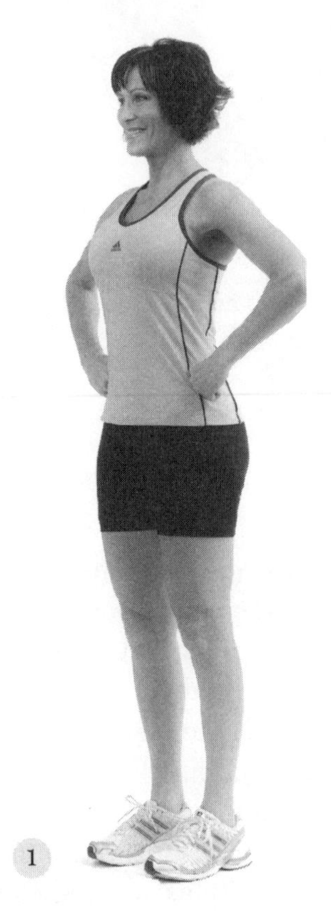

START: Feet wider than hip width apart, chest lifted in a neutral spine alignment, and hands on hips (1).

ACTION: Step forward with your right foot into a long stride (heel strikes the ground), bend both knees and lower your hips until your front thigh and back shin are parallel with the floor, and your knees are bent 90 degrees (2). Pause for one count. Lift hips up by pressing up through your front heel and leg to return to starting position. Repeat with the left leg for 1 repetition.

Repeat 1 to 2 sets × 8 repetitions.

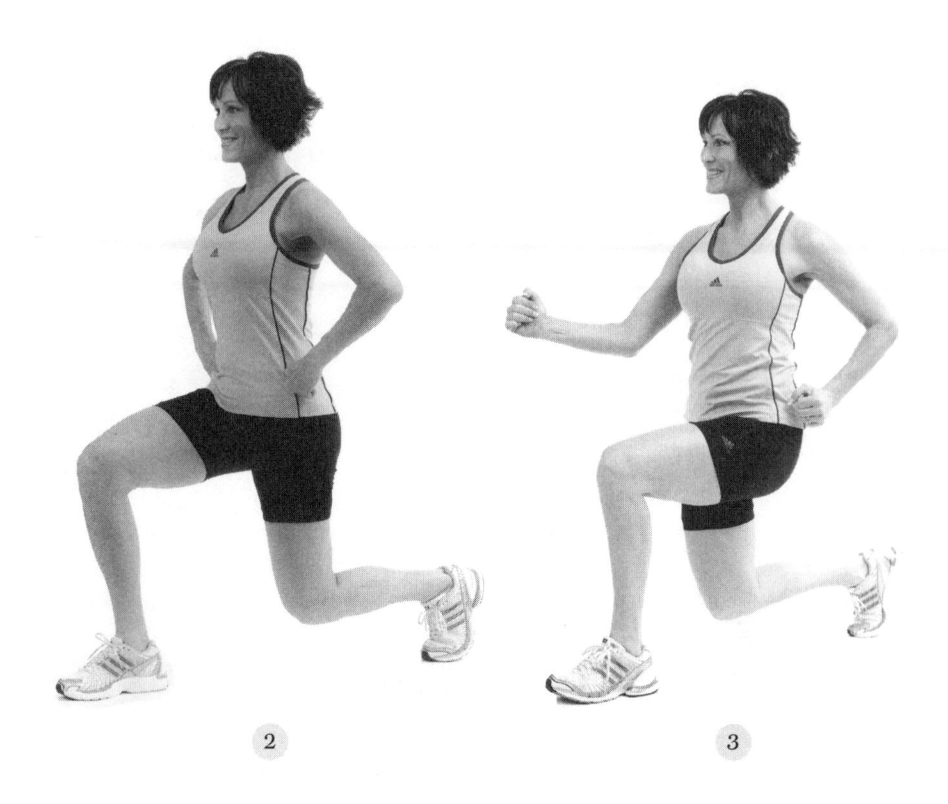

2 3

PROGRESSION: With hands either resting on hips or swinging alongside your body, step forward with the right leg (2) to perform the lunge, return to starting position, then immediately step back with the right leg into a lunge (3); press up through the front heel and lift, then step forward with the right foot to the starting position. Repeat with the left leg. This is 1 repetition.

Repeat 1 set × 8 repetitions on right. Switch and repeat on left.

STEP TOUCH SIDE TO SIDE

Works buttocks (gluteals), quadriceps, and inner and outer thighs

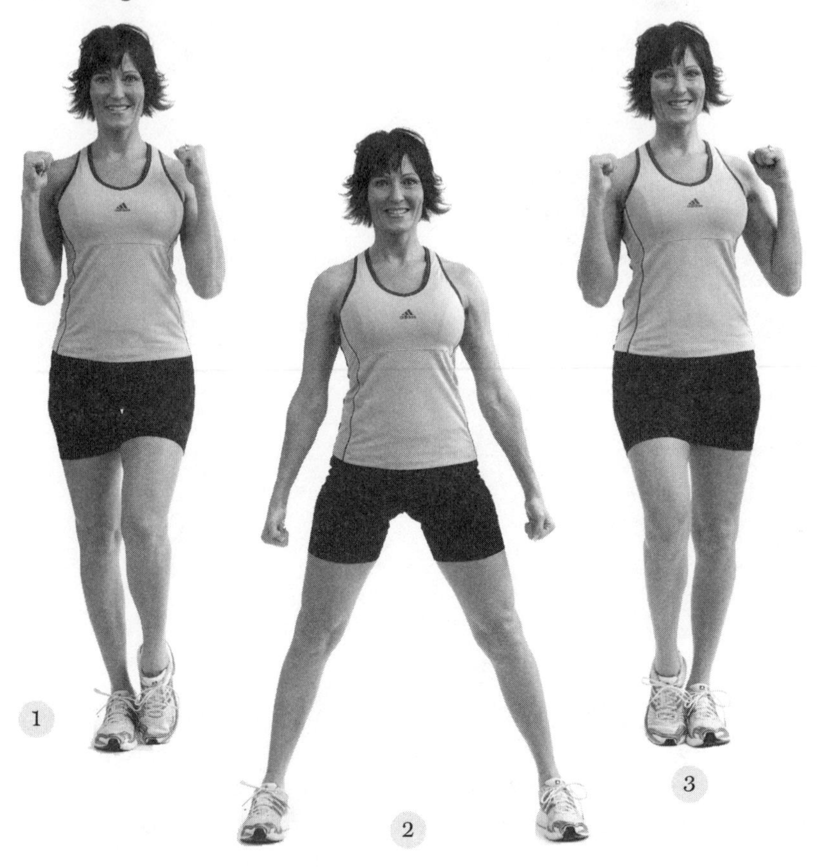

START: Stand on your right foot with your left heel lifted off the floor and knee slightly bent, elbows bent with hands lifted to shoulder level (1).

ACTION: Step to the left into a wide stance and push to extend both arms at your sides (2), bring your right foot in to touch as you bend your elbows and bring your hands back to shoulder level (3), pause to inhale, and return to starting position. Exhale and repeat to the right for 1 repetition.

Repeat 2 sets × 8 repetitions.

WIDE DYNAMIC SQUATS

Works buttocks (gluteals), quadriceps, hamstrings, and inner and outer thighs

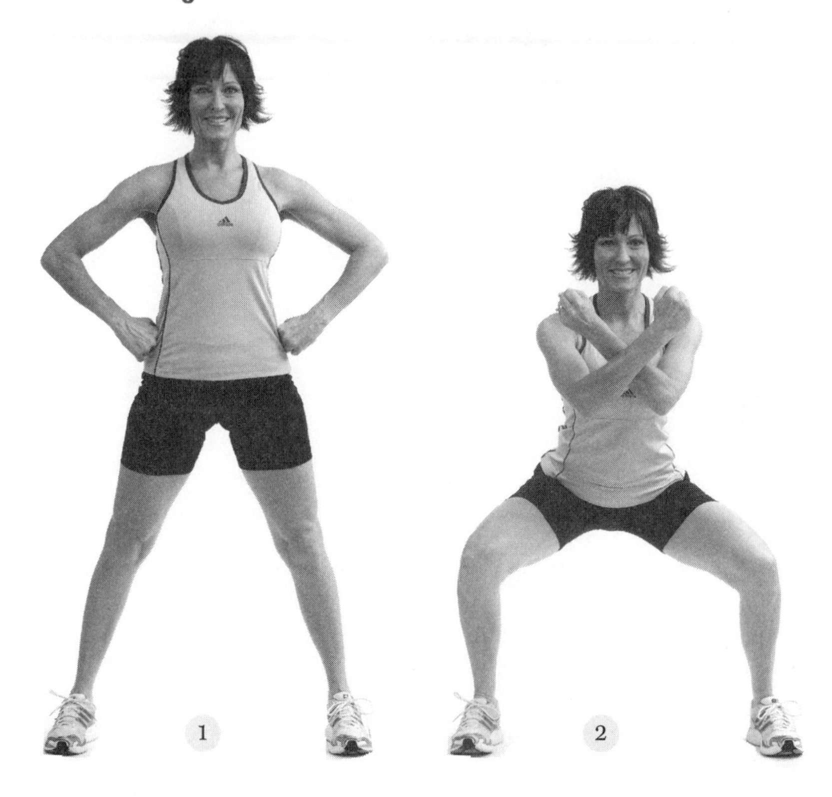

START: Stand in a wide stance, with feet 2 to 3 times wider than your hip width, and feet and knees turned out comfortably and aligned with each other. Stand with a tall, neutral spine—chin level, shoulders down, chest lifted, abdominals pulled in, and buttocks tight. Hands on your hips or top of the thighs (1).

ACTION: Bend your knees and lower your hips straight down into a squat as you bend your elbows and cross your arms in front of your chest (2). Do not lean forward. Pause, and then press up by squeezing your buttocks and inner thighs to rise out of the squat. As you straighten your legs to rise up, slide your left foot in to cross behind your right and pull your elbows back to bring your hands back to your hips (3). Repeat by stepping out with your right foot

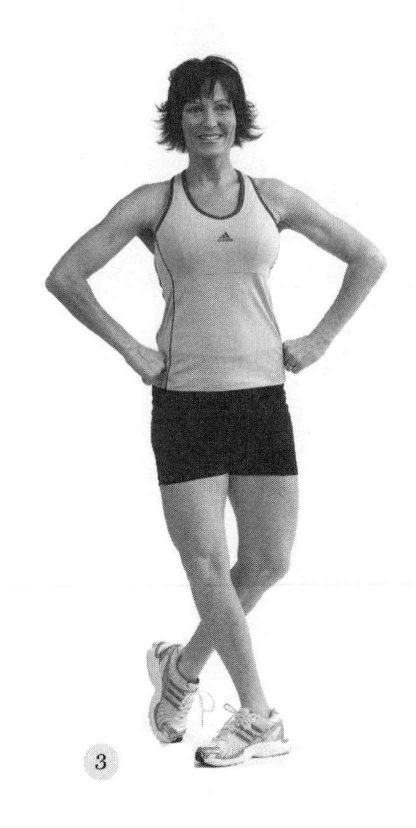

(back to starting position) and lower yourself into a wide squat. Repeat with the right for 1 repetition.

Repeat 2 sets × 8 to 16 repetitions.

PROGRESSION: As you cross your left foot behind your right, march on the spot (right foot, then left); return to wide squat to repeat on the left for 1 repetition.

VARIATION: Perform 2 wide dynamic squats to the right, sliding the left foot in on the first, then crossing it behind the right on the second to march on the spot, then repeat to the left—for 1 repetition. As you squat twice to each side, cross your arms in front of your chest; as you lift up and out of the squat, pull your arms down (elbows back); as you perform the second squat to the right, repeat the chest press; and as you step in or cross behind with your left foot, pull your hands to your hips. Repeat as directed to the left for 1 repetition.

Repeat 2 sets of 8 to 16 repetitions.

THE BEST OF BOTH IN 30 MINUTES

The Newbody 30-minute workout alternates between aerobic and functional strength training, and should be completed with a 1-, 2-, or 3-pound dumbbell in each hand. Aerobic training, by the nature of its name, implies that you will increase your heart and respiratory rate for at least 10 minutes. Functional strength training means that you will be strengthening your muscles by doing exercises that mimic movements and patterns of daily life, such as leaning, lifting, pushing, pulling, lunging, squatting, and twisting. Complete the number of sets and repetitions as directed. It is recommended that you work through each sequence leading with the right leg, then repeat leading with the left (each sequence will be performed twice). Commit 10 minutes to each sequence (aerobic and functional strength) for a complete 20-minute workout, leaving you adequate time for the warm-up and recovery. If you complete it faster, then go through each sequence again.

Aerobic Conditioning

ALTERNATING KNEE LIFT WITH ALTERNATING PUSH/PULL

Works your buttocks (gluteals), quadriceps, deltoids, and biceps

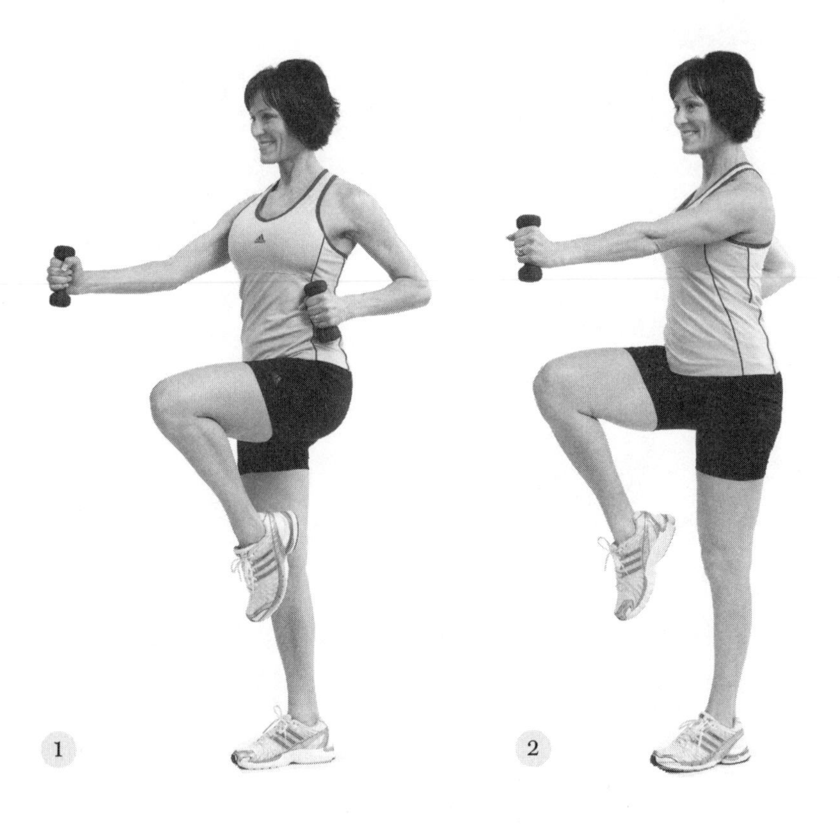

START: Stand tall with feet hip width apart, arms at your sides with elbows bent at about 90 degrees, and a dumbbell in each hand.

ACTION: Step on the right foot to lift the left knee up to hip level as you push your right arm straight out in front, simultaneously pulling your left elbow back behind your body (1). Lower your left knee down to step onto your left foot and lift your right knee up and your left arm forward (2). This is 1 repetition. Repeat alternating

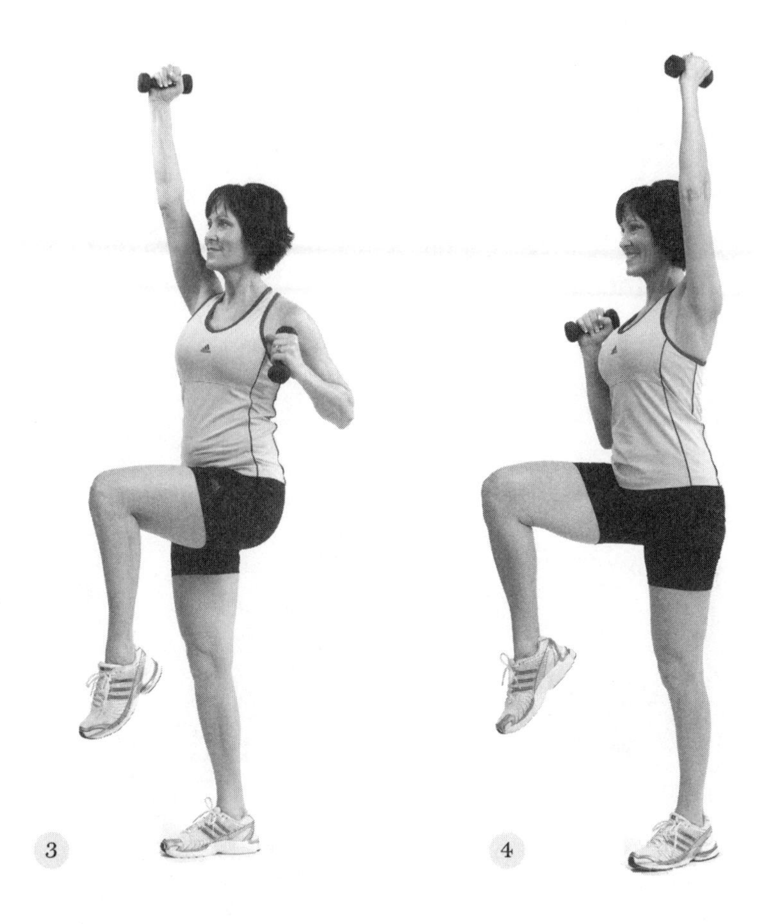

knee lift with arms pushing and pulling in a reciprocal manner, keeping your chest lifted and pushing off the floor to mimic stair climbing.

Repeat 2 to 4 sets × 8 to 16 repetitions.

OPTION: Perform the alternating knee lift bending your elbows and pressing the dumbbells overhead in an alternating manner (3), (4).

Repeat 2 to 4 sets × 8 to 16 repetitions.

CRESCENT LUNGE WITH BENT-OVER SINGLE-ARM ROW

Works buttocks (gluteals), quadriceps, back muscles, rear deltoids, and triceps

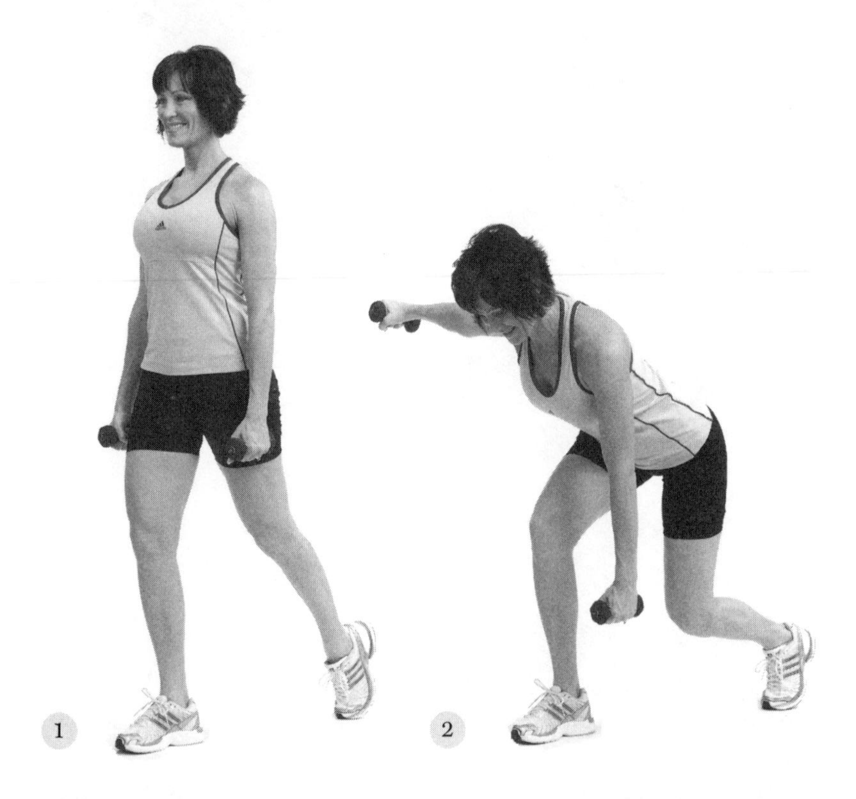

START: Stand with feet hip width apart, step right foot forward into a split stance (moderate stride with back heel lifted off the floor), hands alongside your body with chest lifted, and spine in neutral alignment, with a dumbbell in each hand (1).

ACTION: Bend your knees and lower hips until your front thigh is at 45 degrees and your back shin is approaching parallel with the floor. Lean forward at the hip, maintaining a neutral spine; lift your right arm out to the side and lower your left arm straight down toward the floor (2). Hold the lunge as you bend the left elbow and

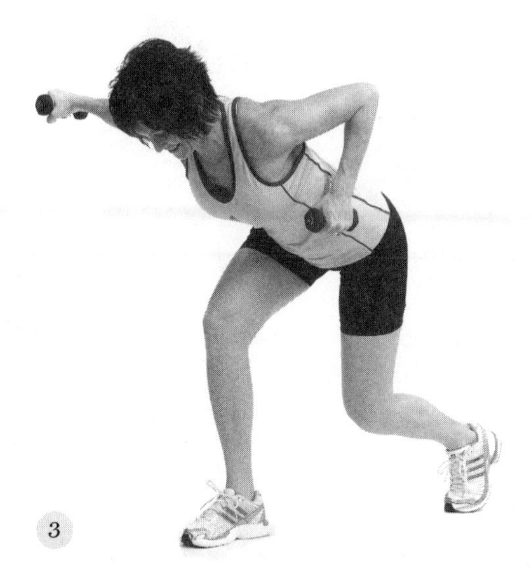

pull the dumbbell upwards until the upper arm is parallel with the floor (3). Lower the left dumbbell, lift your hips upward by pressing through the front heel and leg, lower right arm, and return to starting position. This is 1 repetition.

Repeat 2 to 4 sets × 8 to 16 repetitions. Switch legs and repeat.

PROGRESSION: Repeat the crescent lunge (1), (2), and repeat the single-arm row 3 consecutive times (triple row), then return to starting position and repeat as indicated.

Repeat 4 sets of triple-arm row on each side.

OPTION: Place both dumbbells in one hand to increase the intensity of the row.

GRAPEVINE HEEL LIFT SEQUENCE

Works buttocks (gluteals), hamstrings, and inner and outer thighs

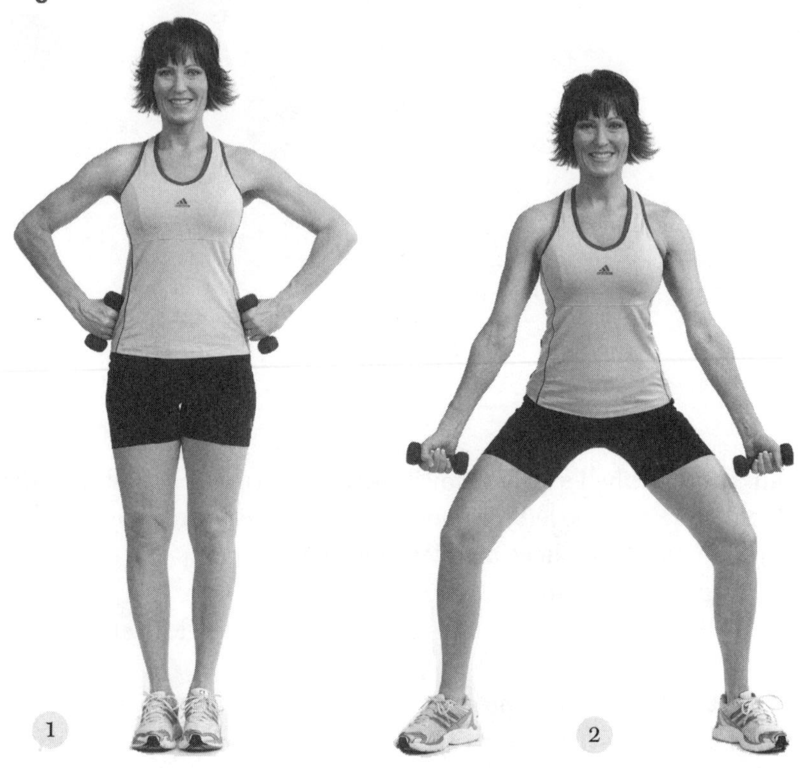

START: Stand with feet together; neutral spine alignment with shoulders back, chest lifted, and elbows bent with hands on hips (1).

ACTION: Step to the left side, pushing off your right foot, and straighten your arms out to your side, squeezing your shoulder blades (2). Step your right foot behind your left (3), then step out to the left with your left foot as you bend your elbows and cross the dumbbells up in front to chest level, (4) then step to the left, lift your right heel up, and bend your left heel up behind (5), squeezing your buttocks as you lift your heel. Repeat to the right. This is 1 repetition.

Repeat 4 to 8 sets of 8 repetitions.

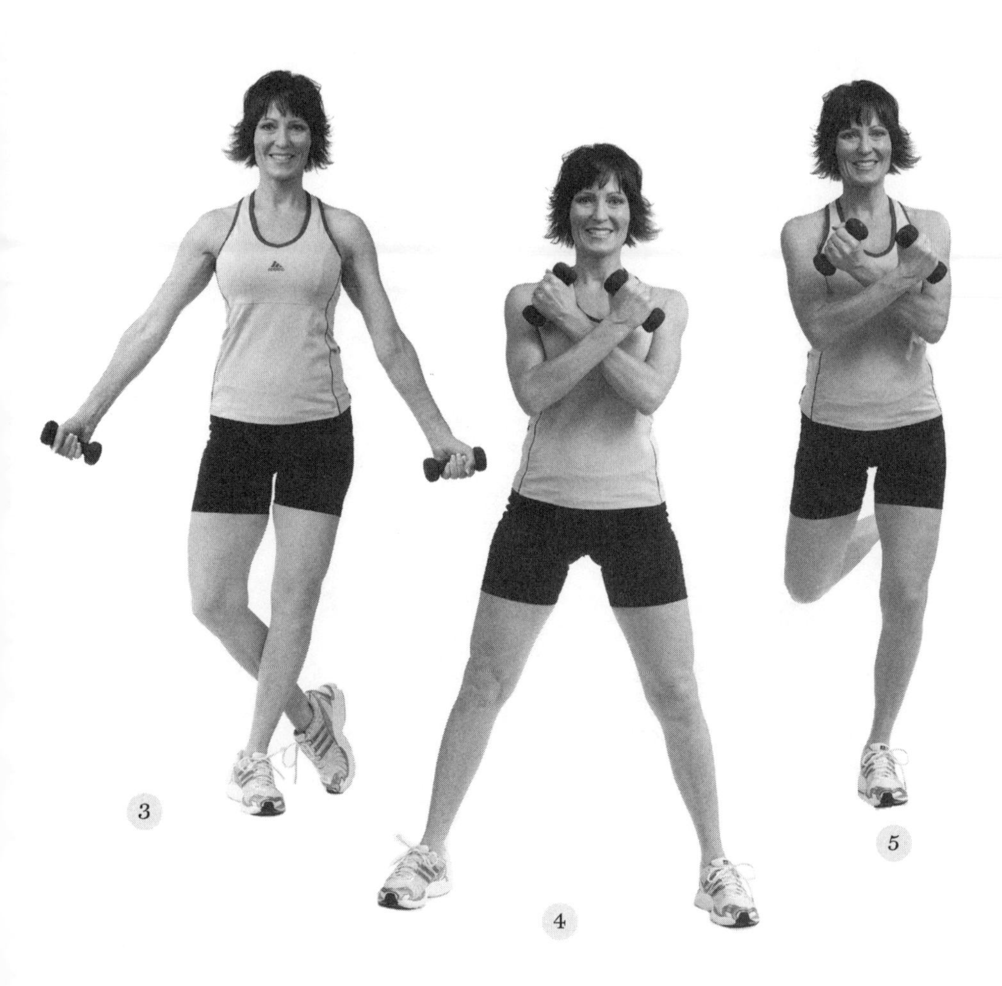

PROGRESSION: Bend your knees as you step out (into a deeper squat) and lower your centre of gravity down to help move your body up as you lift your heels up behind you. Push up through your standing leg as you lift the heel and push-pull the dumbbells to emphasize the movement.

Repeat 2 to 4 sets of 8 to 16 repetitions.

SKATE SEQUENCE

Works buttocks (gluteals) and hamstrings

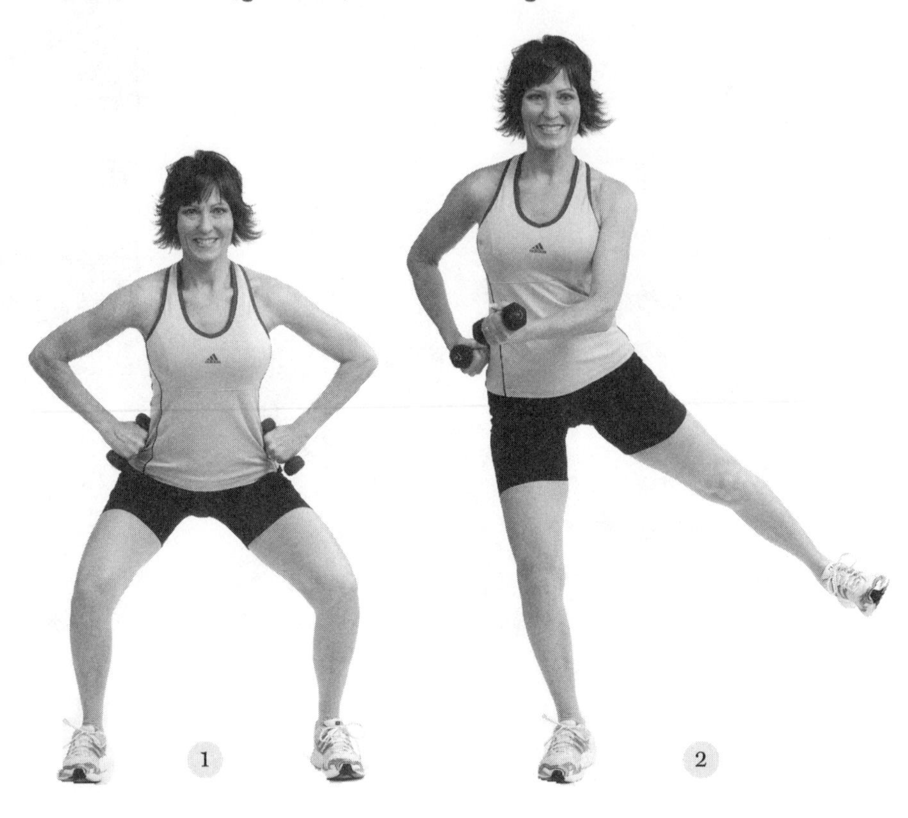

START: Stand in a wide stance or partial squat, with feet 2 times wider than your hip width, and feet and knees turned out comfortably and aligned with each other. Place hands on your hips or together in front of your waist with abdominals pulled in and buttocks tight, chest lifted, and shoulders back (1).

ACTION: Squeeze your butt and bend your knees to lower into a deeper squat, keeping them aligned with your feet, push off your right foot to lift your left leg up off the floor (2), back and out wide to the side (skating action) as you push your left arm up and across the torso, keeping the elbow bent at 45 degrees. Lower the left leg and return to a deeper squat (3) and repeat, pushing off the left foot

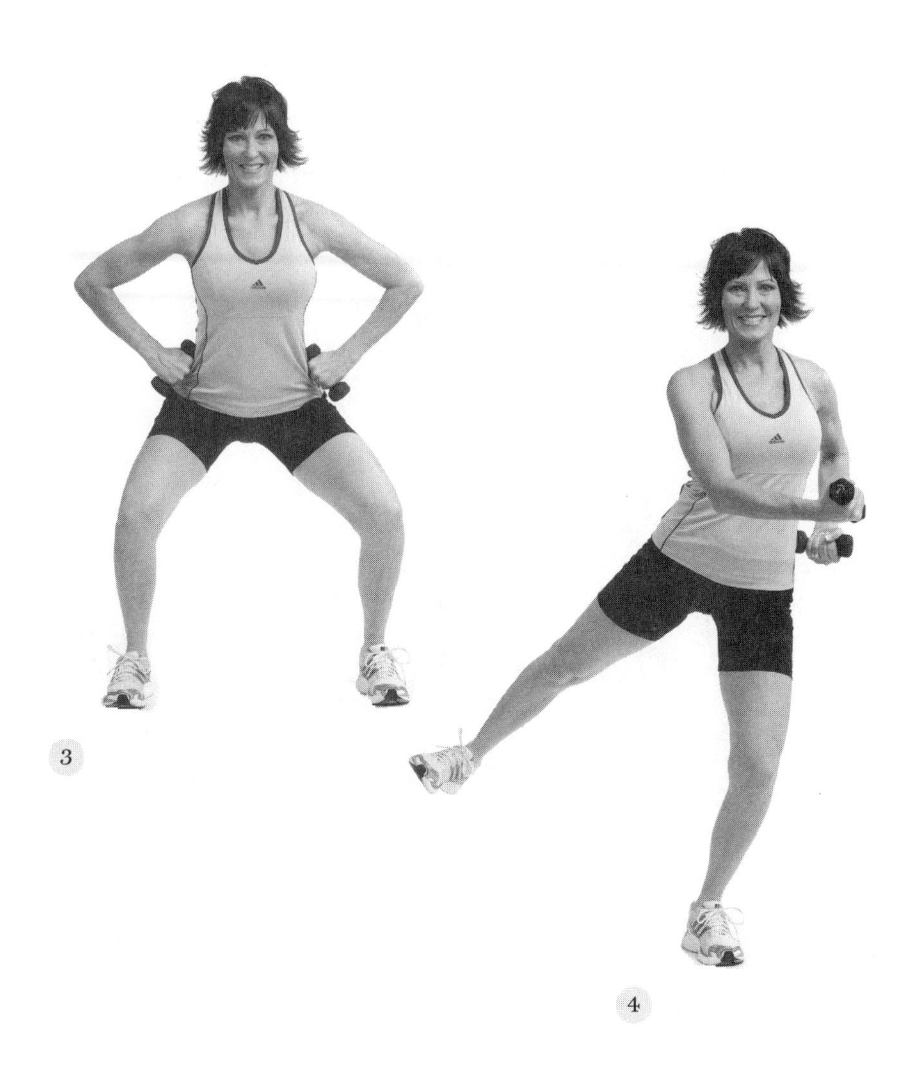
3

4

to lift the right leg (4). This is 1 repetition. Keep your abdominals pulled in and buttocks squeezed tight to maintain a neutral spine. Lean forward at the hip to lift the leg higher in the skating action but do not allow your back to arch.

Repeat 4 sets of 8 to 16 repetitions.

DYNAMIC CURTSY SQUATS

Works buttocks (gluteals), quadriceps, and hamstrings

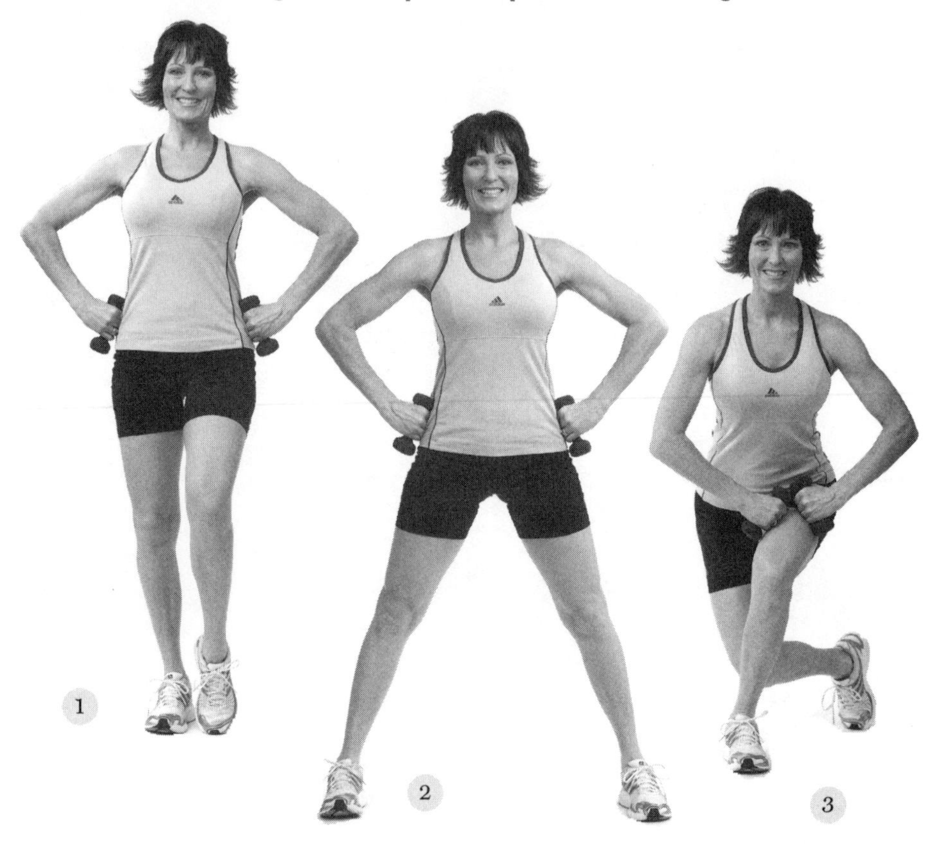

START: Stand with feet together and weight on right foot, left knee slightly bent with heel lifted, and hands on hips with dumbbells in your hand. Keep spine in a neutral alignment, with chest lifted, shoulders down, abdominals pulled in, and buttocks tight (1).

ACTION: Step out to the side with your left foot into a wide stance (2). Step your right foot in and cross it behind the left with the knee turned out slightly and lower your hips down by bending both knees. Pause in a "curtsy" squat for 1 count (3), then lift up and step out with your right foot into a wide stance (2) and repeat the curtsy squat to the right as directed. This is 1 repetition.

Repeat 2 to 4 sets of 8 to 16 repetitions.

Functional Strength

DEAD LIFT AND BENT-OVER ROW SEQUENCE

Works shoulder and back muscles, buttocks (gluteals), and hamstrings

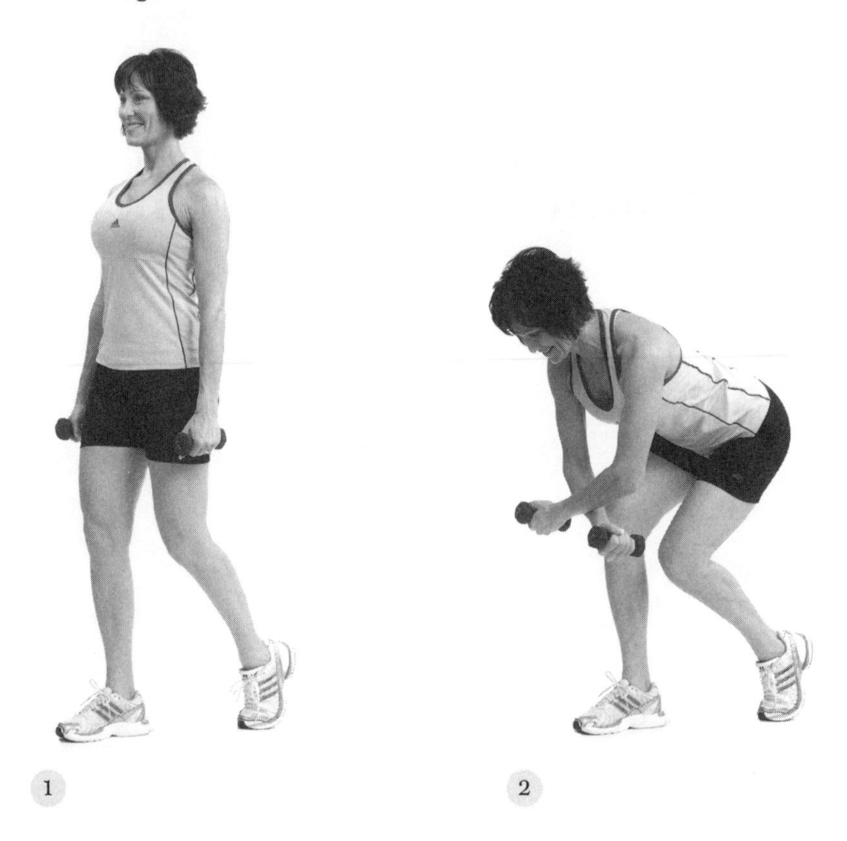

1 2

START: Stand with feet hip width apart and a dumbbell in each hand; palms facing in, shoulders down, abdominals pulled in, buttocks squeezed, and knees slightly bent to maintain a neutral spine. Step back with the left foot to a split stance, heel lifted up (1).

ACTION: Bend your knees and lean forward from the hips as you keep your spine in a neutral alignment until the dumbbells are just below knee level; cross one arm in front of the other, squeezing through the chest, and pause for 1 count (2). Exhale and lift your arms out to the side and up until they are parallel with the floor,

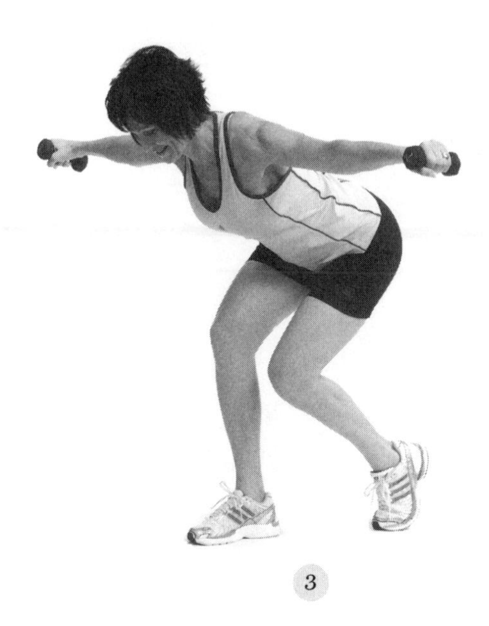

3

squeeze your shoulder blades toward the spine; keep your chin in and aligned with your chest to maintain a neutral spine. Hold for 1 count (3). Lower the dumbbells slowly in front of your knees and lift up to return to starting position (1). Step in with your left leg, move your right leg behind, and repeat. This is 1 repetition.

Repeat 2 to 4 sets of 8 repetitions.

SINGLE-LEG LIFT 'N' EXTEND

Works buttocks (gluteals) and quadriceps

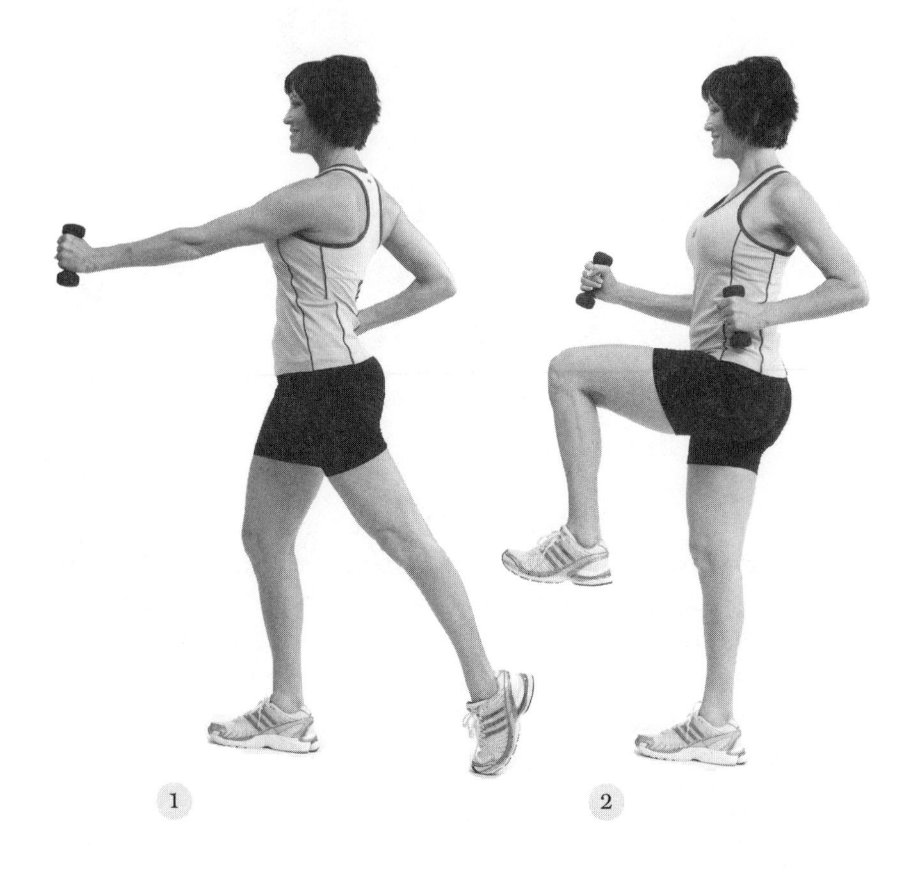

START: Stand with feet hip width apart, left leg extended behind with your heel lifted, left arm pushing forward, and right elbow pulling back, with a dumbbell in each hand (1). Keep your abdominals pulled in, chest lifted, and spine in neutral alignment with your shoulders down, away from your ears.

ACTION: Lift left knee up in front to hip level, bending the knee 90 degrees as you simultaneously pull your left elbow back to bring your left hand to your hip; your right arm pushes forward (2). Squeeze your buttocks and push through your left leg to extend it

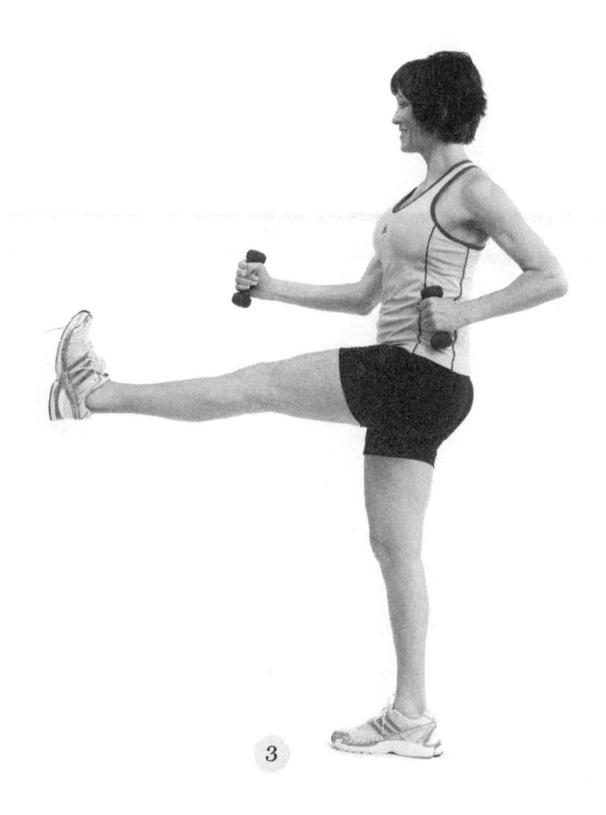

(straighten) it out in front at hip level (3). Pause for 1 count; inhale, and then exhale as you bend the left knee and push it back to the starting position, simultaneously pushing the left arm forward. Pause for 1 count. This is 1 repetition.

Repeat 2 sets of 8 to 16 repetitions. Switch to the other leg and repeat as indicated.

STATIONARY SQUATS WITH ANTERIOR SHOULDER RAISE

Works buttocks (gluteals), quadriceps, hamstrings, abdominals, and deltoids

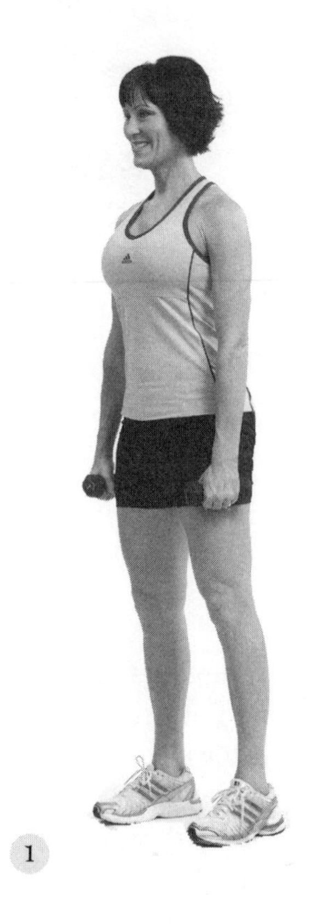

1

START: Stand with feet just wider than hip width, knees slightly bent and aligned over toes, and arms at sides. Keep spine in neutral alignment, with chest lifted, and hold one dumbbell in each hand (1).

ACTION: Bend at the knees to lower your hips back and toward the floor until your thighs are at least at a 45-degree angle (halfway to parallel) with the floor. Push your arms out in front and up to

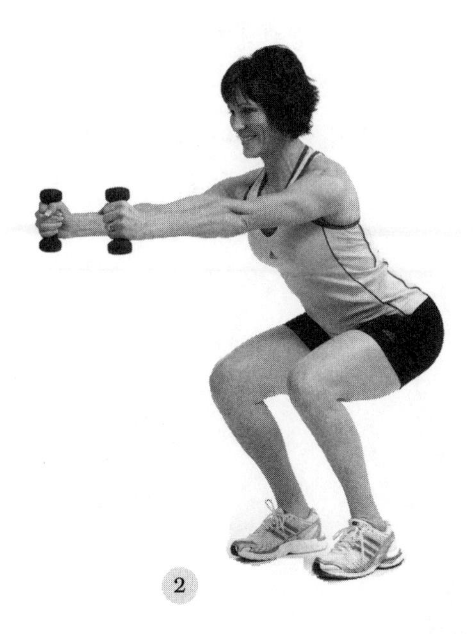

shoulder level (2). Pause for 1 to 2 counts and inhale. As you exhale, return to the starting position by pushing up through your legs. Lower your arms at your sides. This is 1 repetition.

Repeat 2 to 4 sets of 8 to 16 repetitions.

OPTION: Place your arms at your sides and perform the squat as indicated for less intensity; this makes for a greater balance challenge.

DEAD LIFT WITH REAR LEG LIFT

Works buttocks (gluteals), quadriceps, hamstrings, and back muscles

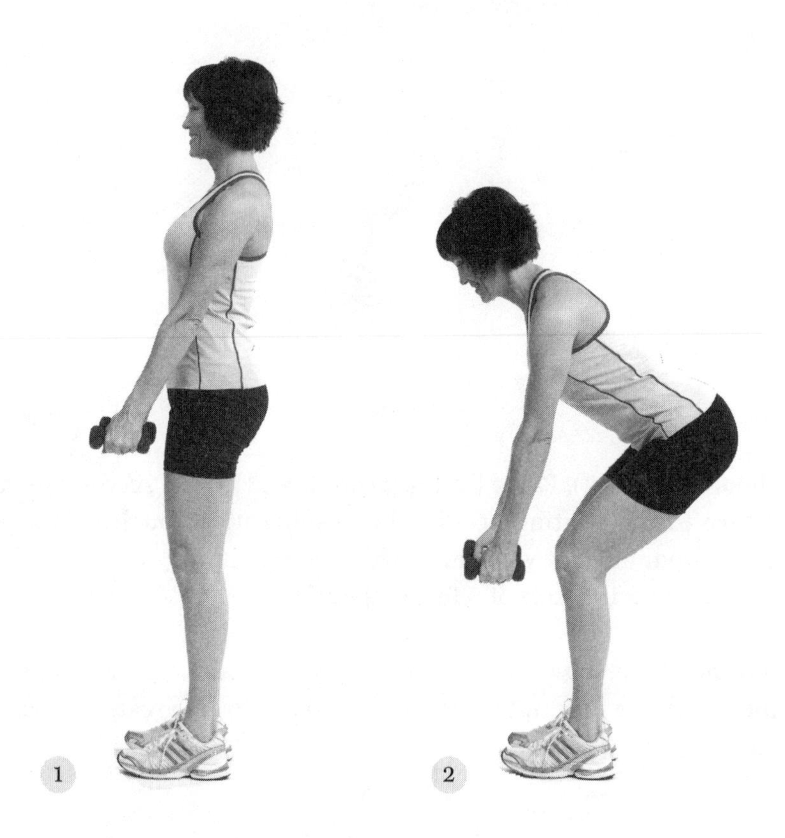

START: Stand with feet hip width apart and arms straight at your sides with palms facing in, a dumbbell in each hand. Keep your buttocks squeezed, abdominals pulled in, chest lifted, and spine in neutral alignment; keep your shoulders down away from your ears (1).

ACTION: Bend your knees and hinge (lean) forward from the hips as you keep your spine in neutral, until the dumbbells are just below knee level (2). Pause to inhale for 1 count, then exhale as you lift the

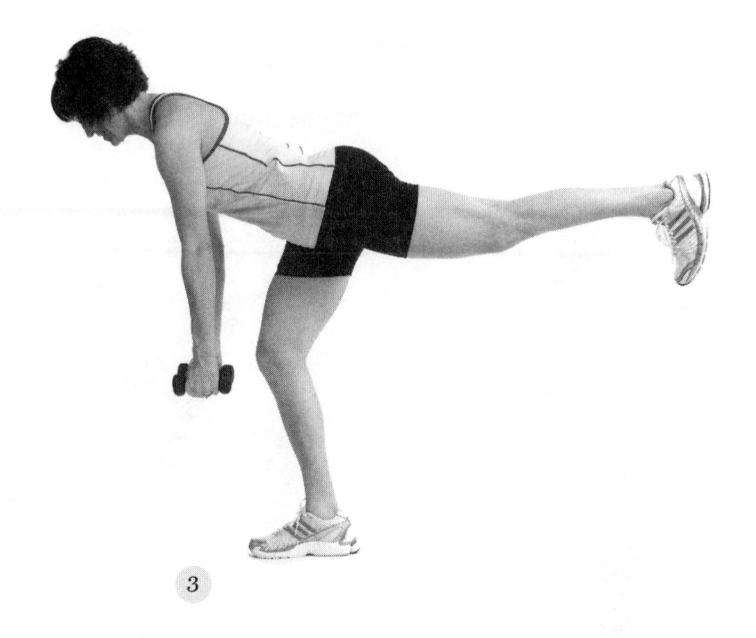

left leg until your heel is level with your hip (3). Pause for 1 count. Inhale, lower your back foot down to (2); exhale and press up to return to standing/starting position (1). This is 1 repetition.

Repeat 2 sets of 8 to 16 repetitions. Switch legs and repeat as indicated.

OPTION: Repeat the dead lift without the rear leg lift (1), (2), to minimize intensity. Repeat 4 sets of 8 to 16 repetitions.

SINGLE-LEG SQUAT ON THE SPOT

Works buttocks (gluteals), quadriceps, hamstrings, deltoids, and chest

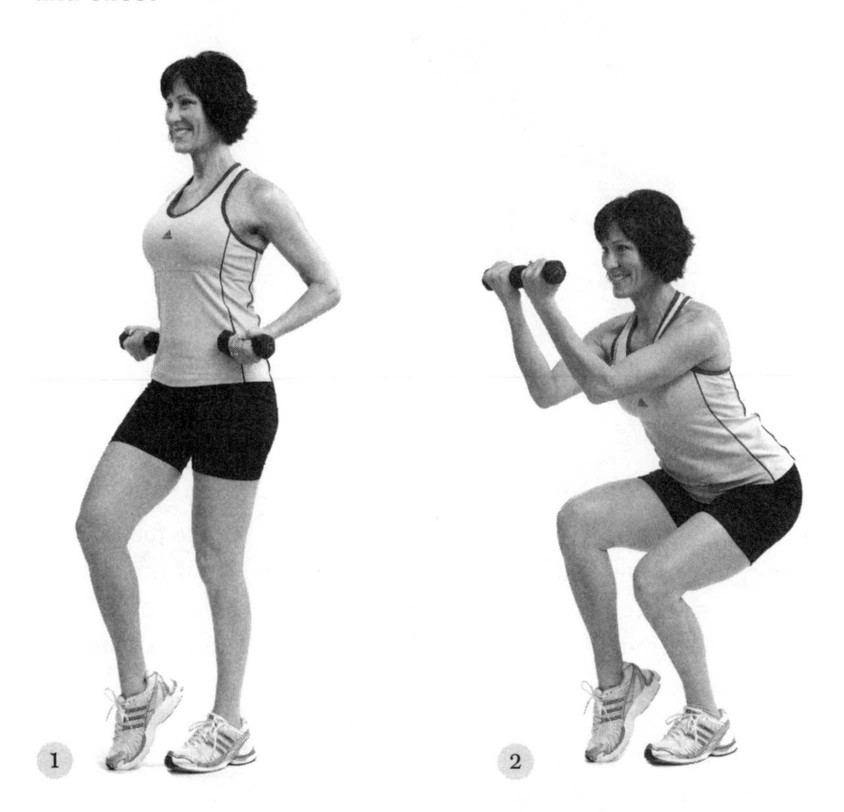

START: Stand with feet just wider than hip width, knees slightly bent and aligned over your toes, with a dumbbell in each hand and your hands on your hips. Keep your spine in neutral, with your chest lifted, abdominals pulled in, and buttocks squeezed tight as you transfer your bodyweight onto your left leg and lift your right heel off the floor (1).

ACTION: Bend at the knees to lower your hips back and down toward the floor until your thighs are at least at a 45-degree angle (halfway parallel with the floor); you should eventually manage to get them parallel. Push and press the dumbbells up toward the ceiling until your elbows are chest level, or your upper arms are almost parallel with the floor (2). Pause for 1 count. Exhale, press up to return to starting position by pushing down into the left heel and pressing up through the left leg. This is 1 repetition.

Repeat 2 to 4 sets of 8 to 16 repetitions. Switch sides and repeat as indicated.

PLIÉ SQUAT WITH TORSO TWISTS

Works buttocks (gluteals), quadriceps, hamstrings, inner and outer thighs, abdominals/core, and back muscles

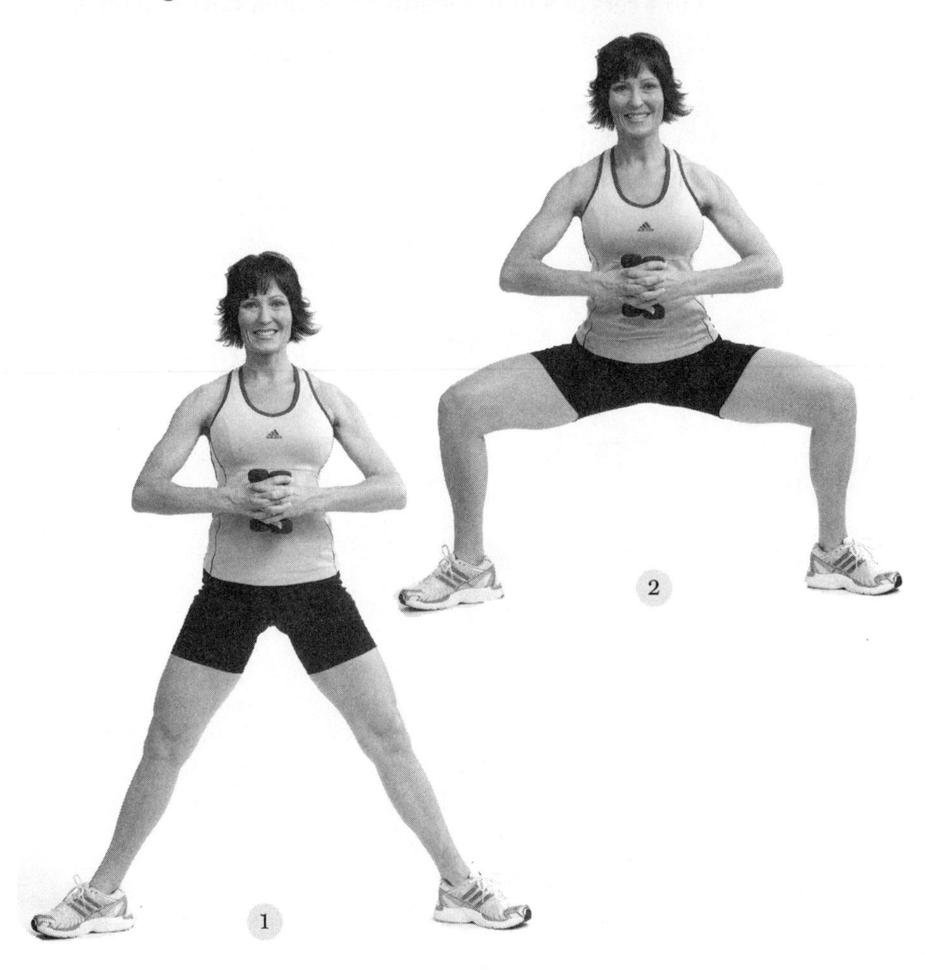

START: Stand in a wide stance, with feet 2 to 3 times wider than hip width apart, and feet and knees turned out comfortably and aligned with each other. Stand with a tall, neutral spine—chin level, shoulders down, chest lifted, abdominals pulled in, and buttocks tight. Brace the dumbbells in your hands; interlace your fingers to hold the dumbbells in front of your body at waist level (1).

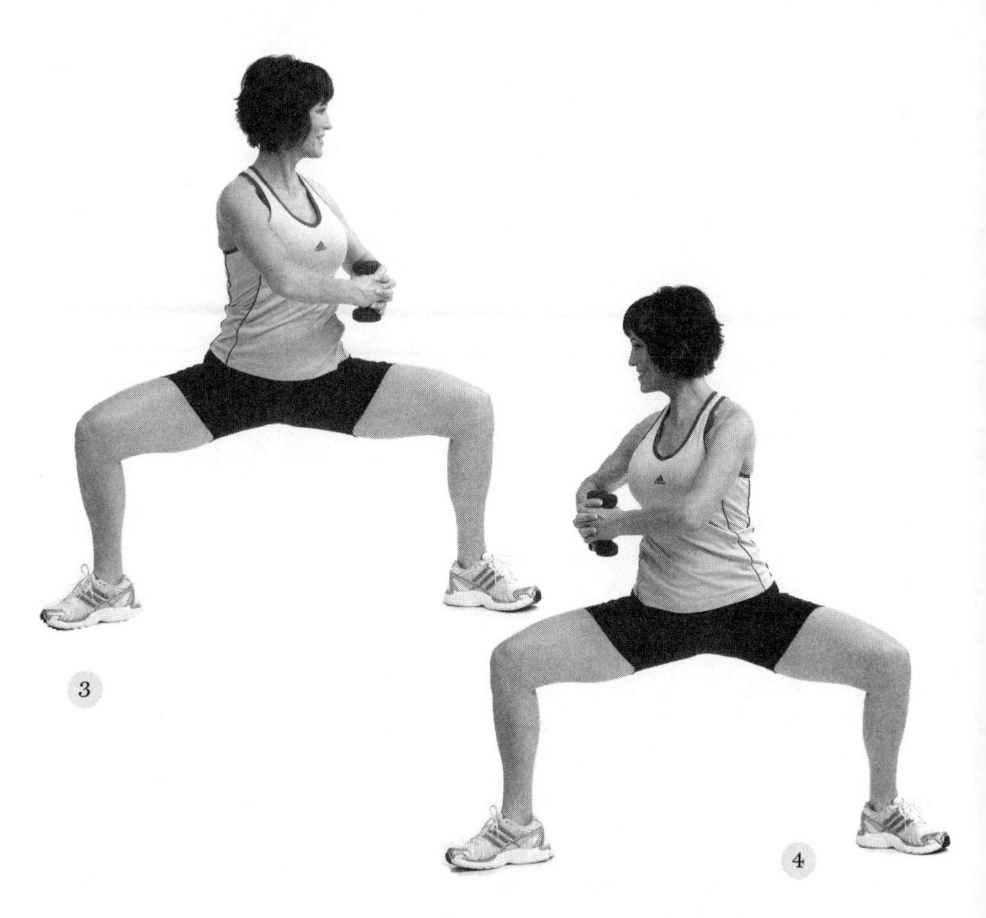

ACTION: Bend your knees and lower your hips straight down into a plié squat (2). Do not lean forward. Hold this position, then turn your torso to the left (3), return to the centre, turn to the right (4), return to the centre; then press up by squeezing your buttocks and inner thighs to rise out of the squat and return to starting position (1).

PROGRESSION: Repeat the plié squat as indicated; perform 4 to 8 torso twists (left then right); return to the centre, then to the starting position for 1 set.

Repeat: perform the torso twists right to left for 1 set. Repeat 1 to 2 sets of 4 to 8 repetitions.

VARIATION: As you straighten your legs to rise up, slide your right foot in to meet your left. Repeat the plié squat with torso twist as indicated, and as you straighten your legs to rise up, slide your left foot in to meet your right. This is 1 repetition.

Repeat 2 sets of 4 to 8 repetitions.

The Recovery: Range of Motion and Flexibility

The recovery is as important as the workout. Stretching your muscles increases flexibility, helps to maintain a healthy range of movement around the joints, and aids recovery after exercise. Stretching increases blood flow to and from the working muscles, delivering nutrients for muscle repair and growth, as well as helping to soothe muscle soreness following exercise. Take the extra time to learn how to stretch correctly (as I have shown you), but once you are familiar with this stretch routine, you will be able to complete all the standing stretches within 7 minutes. Learn the floor stretches too because they are very effective for advancing your flexibility—try those stretches before you go to bed or first thing in morning before you get out of bed. The more you stretch the better you will feel, so feel free to repeat any or all of them more than 1 repetition each side.

QUADRICEPS STRETCH

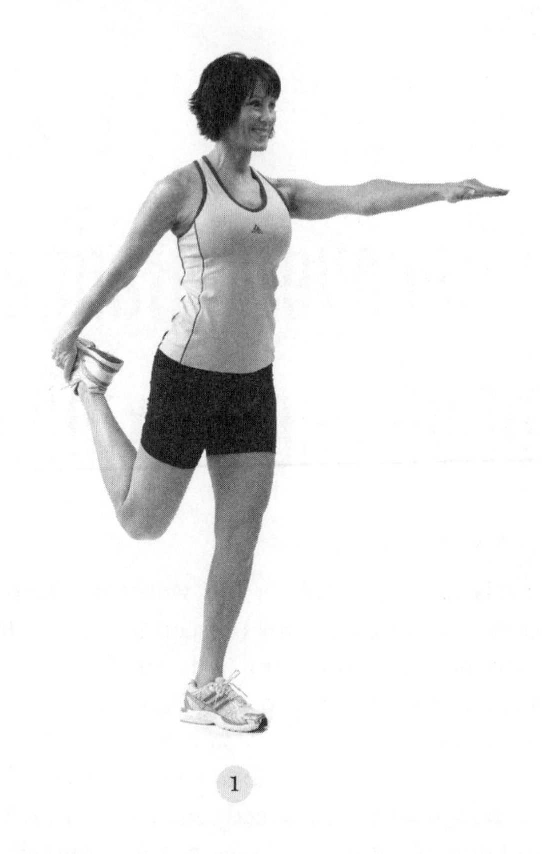

1

START: Stand tall with feet hip width apart and left hand on your hip or lifted out in front or to the side to help you maintain your balance.

ACTION: Bend your right knee and lift your right heel up behind you; reach back and grasp it with your right hand. Keeping your right knee pointing downward, gently pull your heel toward your hip without leaning forward or back, to feel a stretch down the front of the right thigh to the knee (1). Keep your abdominals pulled in and squeeze your buttocks and inner thighs to help maintain proper alignment and balance.

Hold the stretch for 1 to 2 breaths, 3 to 5 seconds. Lower your leg. Repeat on the other side.

CALF AND CHEST STRETCH

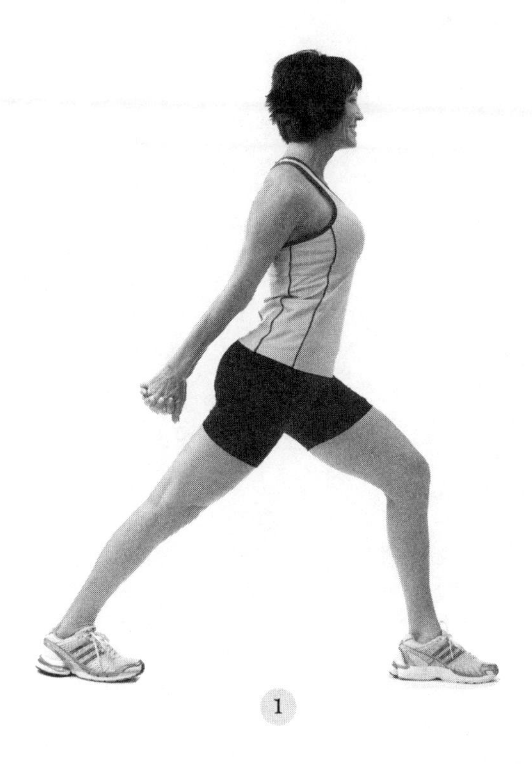

1

START: Stand with feet hip width apart. Step back in a long stride with your right leg. Interlace your fingers behind your back.

ACTION: Gently press your back heel toward the floor as you straighten your back leg. Bend your front knee and hold the stretch (1) for 1 to 2 breaths, 3 to 5 counts. Lift your chest and your arms away from your back as you breathe. Return to start. Repeat on the other side.

LATERAL BODY STRETCH

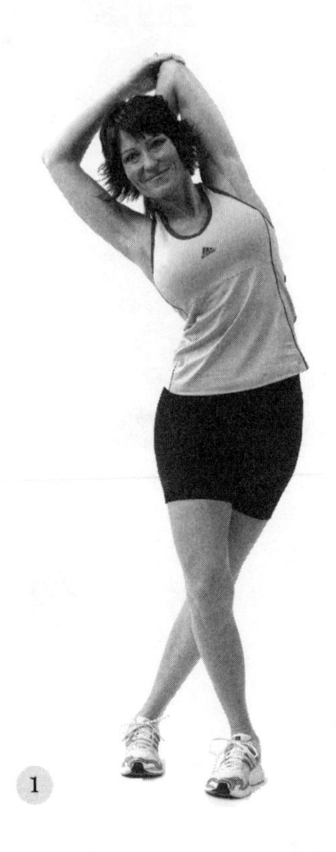

START: Stand on your right foot and cross your left foot behind; keep your feet wider than shoulder width apart and your toes pointed forward. Place your right hand on your hip for balance as you lift your left arm up overhead.

ACTION: Bend your left elbow and assist the stretch by gently pulling the elbow over to the right side with your right hand. Lean over toward the right side to feel a stretch along the left side of your trunk, hip, and thigh (1). Hold the stretch for 1 to 2 breaths, 3 to 5 seconds; inhale to return to starting position and repeat the stretch again on the same side. Repeat on the other side.

UPPER BACK AND SHOULDER STRETCH

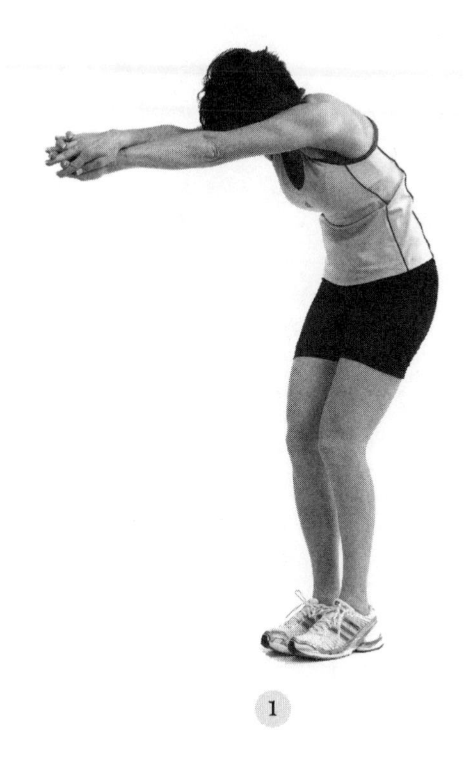

1

START: Stand with feet side by side (or hip width apart for greater stability), knees bent, abdominals pulled in, arms out in front with palms inward (or forearms crossed), and fingers interlaced together.

ACTION: Exhale as you round your middle and lower back and reach your arms out in front of you. Hold the stretch for 1 to 2 breaths (1); inhale as you release. Return to start. Repeat, crossing arms over the other way.

STANDING HAMSTRING STRETCH

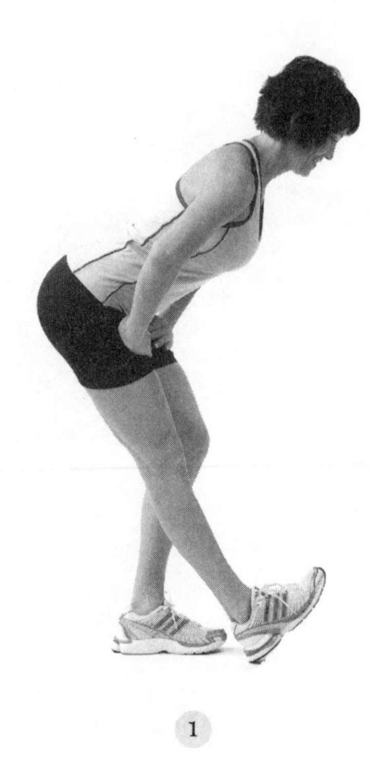

1

START: Stand with feet hip width apart. Place your right heel straight out in front of you, with your toes pulled up toward the ceiling.

ACTION: Lean forward from the hips, maintaining a tall, neutral spine, and bend the left knee slightly. Balance yourself by placing both hands on your thighs. Lift the toes on your right foot up toward the ceiling (1). Hold for 1 breath, stand up and repeat on the same side, reaching down and across to the outside of the foot with your left hand. Hold the stretch for 1 breath, and return to start. Switch legs. Repeat on the other side.

HIP FLEXOR STRETCH

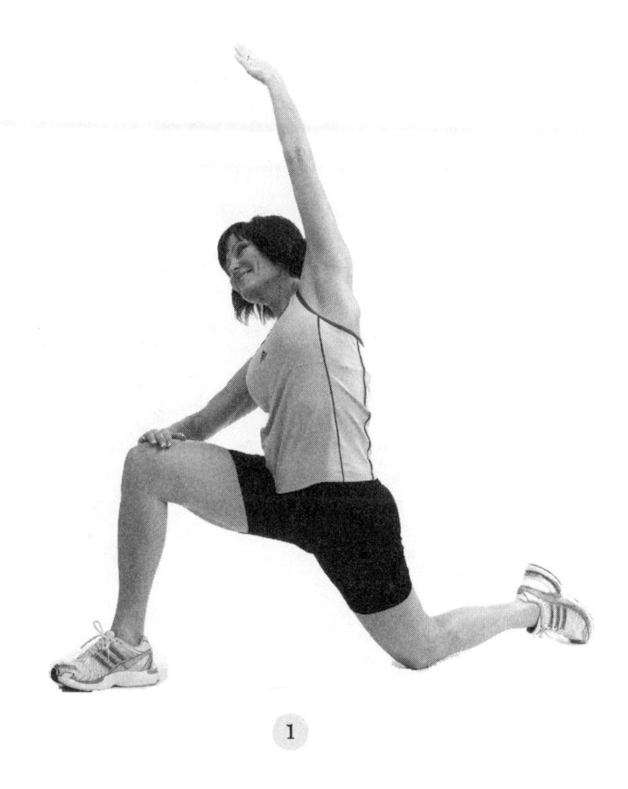

1

START: Stand with feet hip width apart. Step back in a long stride with your left leg and lower your back knee toward the floor; keep your right hand resting on your right thigh.

ACTION: As you pull in your abdominals, tuck your tailbone under, squeeze your buttocks, gently press your hips forward, and lift your chest. Exhale as you press against your front thigh with your right hand and lift your left arm up and laterally overhead toward the right side (1). Hold for 3 to 5 counts and breathe. Repeat on the other side.

OPTION: To intensify the stretch, lift the left knee to straighten the back leg.

INNER THIGH, HAMSTRING, AND BUTTOCK STRETCH

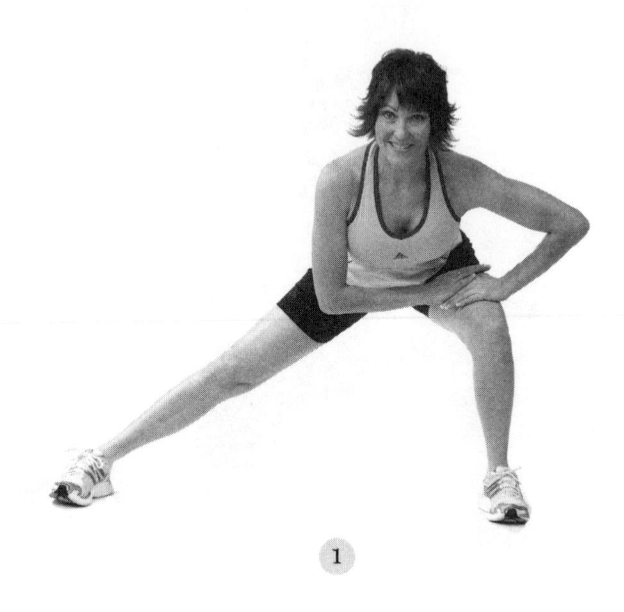

START: Stand in a wide stance, with feet 3 times wider than your hip width apart, and toes forward, weight evenly distributed, and hands on your hips.

ACTION: Bend your left knee and lean forward as you lower your hips back and down. Place your hands on your left thigh to support yourself (1), or lower your right hand to the floor to feel a deeper stretch. Keep your chest lifted and back in neutral. Hold the stretch for 1 to 2 breaths. Return to start. Repeat on the other side.

SEATED SPINAL TWIST

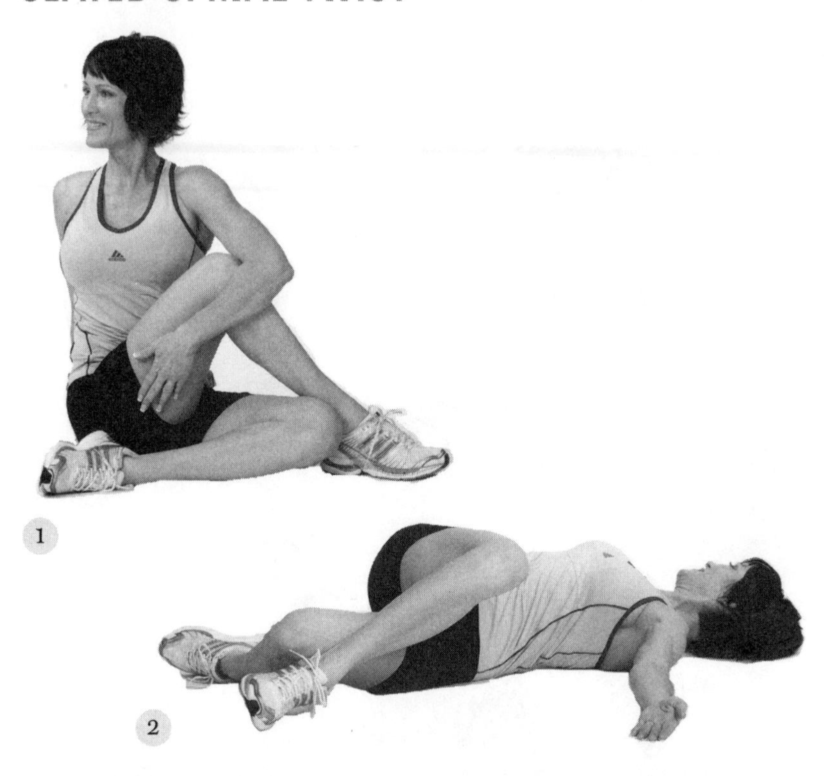

START: Sit on the floor or mat with your left foot tucked under you and your right foot placed over the top of your left leg and flat on the floor. Grasp the right knee with both hands; lift your chest and sit up tall in a neutral position.

ACTION: Inhale and gently twist (rotate) your torso toward your right thigh by pulling with your left hand, while supporting yourself in a tall position with your right hand on the floor behind you (1). Breath in. Exhale and ease off with your left hand, and then repeat again. Return to start, switch legs, and repeat.

OPTION: Lie on your back with both knees bent, your right foot tucked under the left knee and your arms out to the side with palms facing up (2). Hold the stretch for 1 to 2 breaths. Breathe in and repeat on the other side.

SEATED HAMSTRING AND OUTER THIGH STRETCH

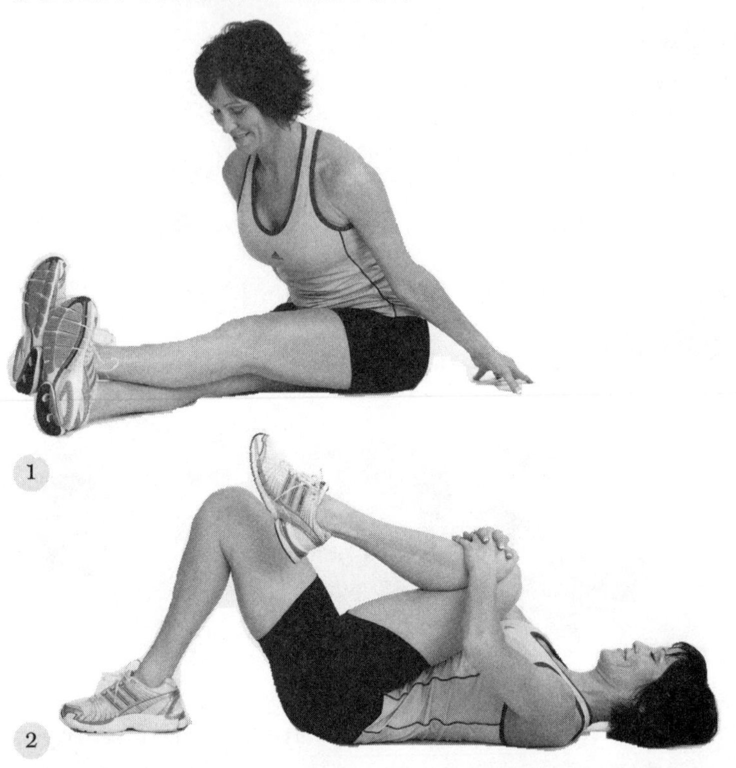

START: Begin in a seated position on the floor, with both legs extended straight out in front of you and toes pointed up; cross the left leg over the right leg. Place your hands behind your hips with fingers away.

ACTION: Inhale and lean forward from your hips with a straight spine (1). Hold for 1 to 2 breaths. Breathe in and repeat, reaching your right hand across to the outside of your left ankle; exhale and hold. Switch legs and repeat.

OPTION: Lie on your back, bending both knees, and bring one or both of them toward your chest with your hands assisting the stretch (2). As you exhale, slowly draw your knees in closer to feel a greater stretch. Inhale as you release and repeat. Repeat on the other side.

BACK "CAT" STRETCH

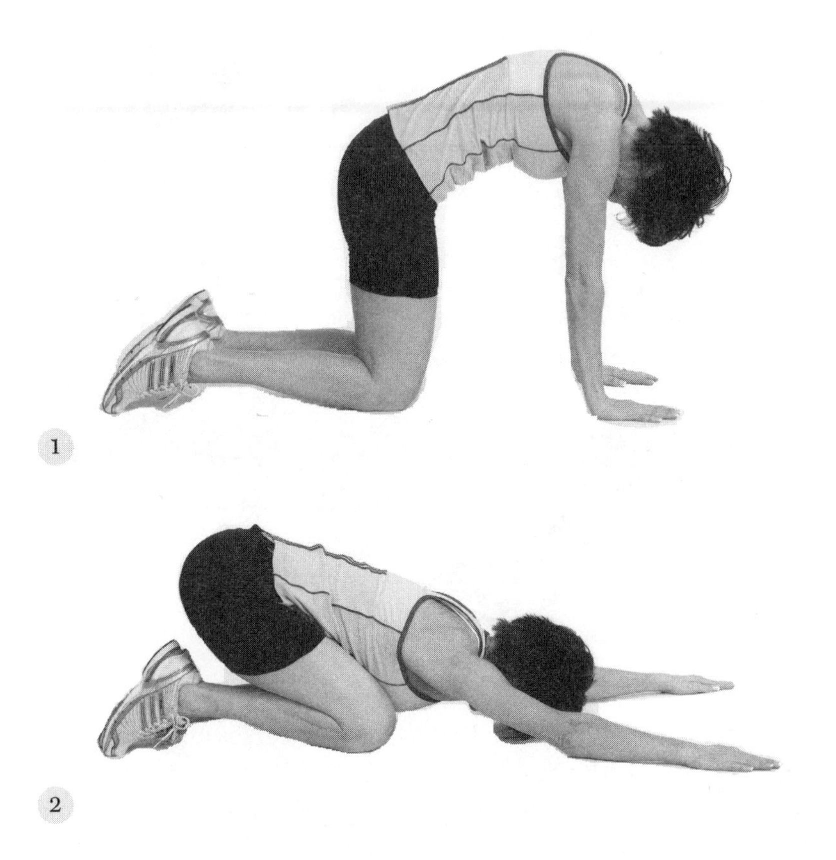

START: Kneel with your hands shoulder width apart and knees hip width apart.

ACTION: Tuck your chin in toward your chest and your tailbone under as you pull your abdominals up and in to round your back and stretch your lower, middle, and upper spine. Hold as you exhale (1); inhale as you release to starting position and repeat.

OPTION: Reach to straighten out your arms in front of you, exhale, and sit your hips back onto your heels while resting your forehead on the floor and your chest on your thighs (2). Exhale as you hold the stretch; inhale as you release and return to starting position. Repeat.

SEATED HIP-OPENER STRETCH

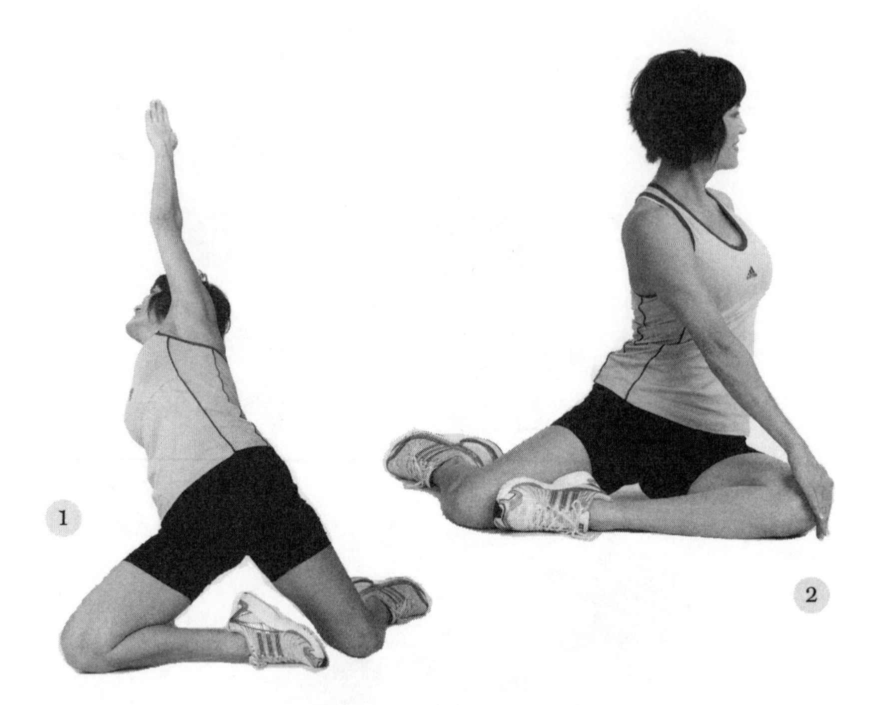

START: Sit on the ground with knees bent 90 degrees and lowered to your right side with your back knee in line with your front heel. Place your right hand behind you to support you in a tall seated position. Keep your abdominals pulled in.

ACTION: Press down into your back hand and lift your hips up off the ground. Squeeze your buttocks to move your hips farther forward and then sweep your left arm across and upwards, following with your eyes, as you exhale (1). Hold the stretch for 2 counts as you inhale; exhale and release; return to starting position. Bring both knees to other side and repeat.

OPTION: Remain sitting with chest lifted and left hand behind your back to help support your spine in a tall, seated position while rotating your torso to the left and assisting the stretch with your right hand pressing against your right knee (2). Hold the stretch for 2 counts as you inhale; exhale and return. Repeat on the other side.

SPINAL EXTENSION STRETCH

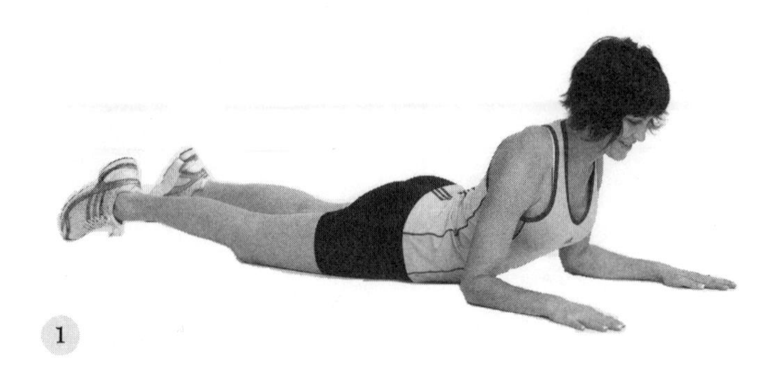

START: Lie face down on the floor or mat and bend your elbows, bringing them alongside your torso at about shoulder width, with palms facing down and chin in to maintain alignment.

ACTION: Exhale as you press up onto your forearms (1) or hands to extend your spine upward. Keep your shoulders down away from your ears and squeeze your buttocks to stabilize your lower back. Pause at the top to breathe in and, as you exhale, lower yourself back to the starting position.

Repeat 3 to 5 times.

Newbody Extra Strength A: Arms, Shoulders, Upper Back, and Chest

The Newbody Extra Strength A routine targets the area for women that has the greatest opportunity for strengthening because this is where women are most weak—in their upper body. Women typically focus on toning their butt and legs; however, a strong and shapely upper body is as important for looks and for function (pushing, pulling, lifting, and carrying) and for maintaining a healthy back. These fabulous four exercises target the arms, shoulders, upper back, and chest while incorporating lower body for a whole-body 15-minute extra strength challenge.

INTENSE SQUAT WITH REAR ARM RAISE

Works near deltoids, triceps, mid back, abdominals and buttocks (gluteals), and quadriceps

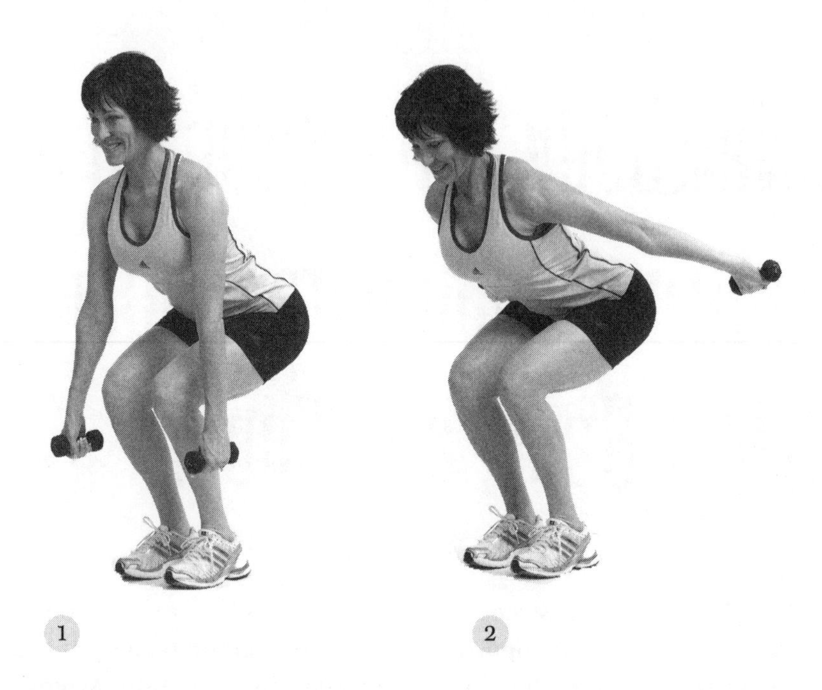

START: Stand with spine in neutral with feet together (or hip width apart for greater balance) and arms alongside your body, palms facing in and holding dumbbells. Squeeze your buttocks, and lower into a squat by bending your knees and pushing your hips back and down. Lean forward slightly, keeping your chest lifted (1).

ACTION: Hold the squat as you push both arms straight back and out wide with your palms facing to the back (2). Pause for 1 or 2 counts as you inhale. Exhale as you lower your arms down to your sides, and push up by pressing into your heels to return to standing; lower yourself back to the starting position (1) and repeat as indicated.

Repeat 2 to 4 sets of 8 repetitions.

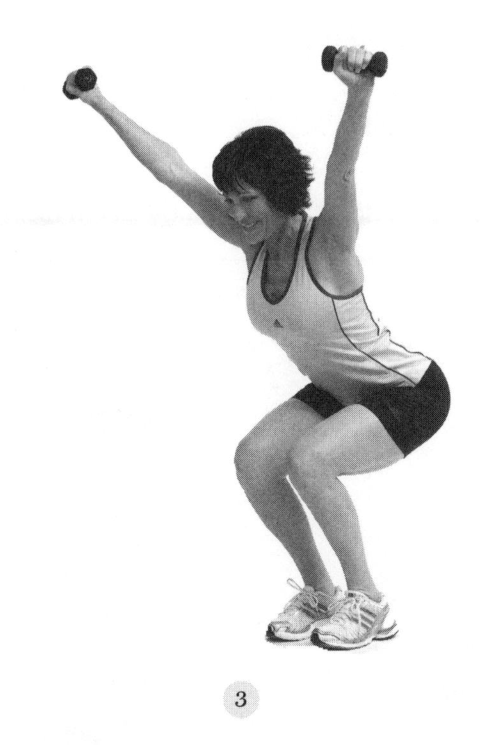

3

PROGRESSION: Repeat the squat (1) and lift both arms up in front overhead with palms facing toward the floor (3). Pause for 1 count; lower the dumbbells toward the floor alongside your outer thighs; push up to return to standing.

Repeat 2 to 4 sets of 8 repetitions

SINGLE BACKWARD/FORWARD LUNGE WITH CROSS-BODY CURL

Works biceps, abdominals, buttocks (gluteals), quadriceps, and hamstrings

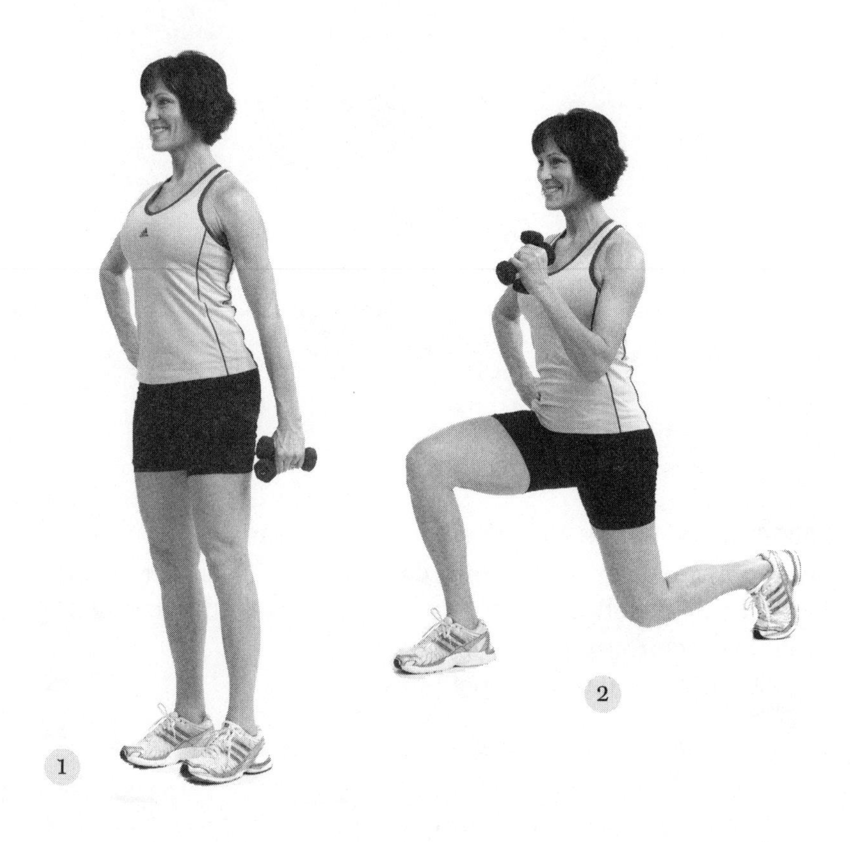

START: Stand with feet hip width apart, right hand on hip, and left arm alongside your body, with one or both dumbbells in your left hand. Chest should be lifted and spine should be in neutral alignment (1).

ACTION: Step backward with the left foot into a long stride; lift your back heel off the floor. Lower your hips until your front thigh and back shin are parallel with the floor, with both knees bent at a

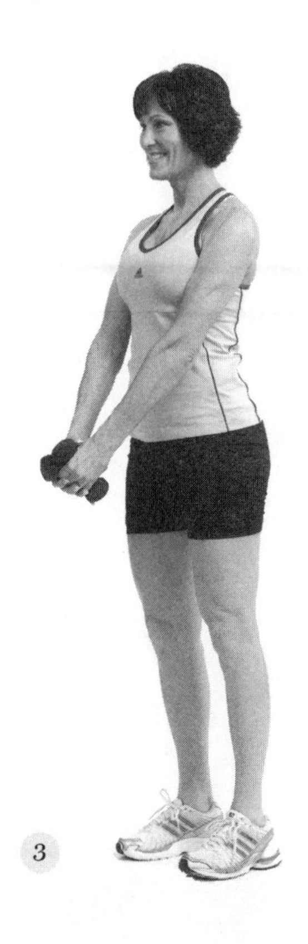
3

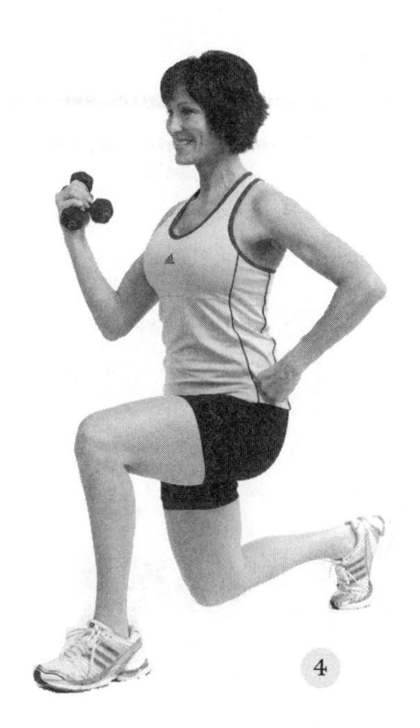
4

90-degree angle. As you lower your hips, bend your left elbow and lift the dumbbells up to shoulder level (2). Pause for 1 count. Lower the dumbbell, lift your hips upward by pressing through the front leg, and step your left foot forward to return to the starting position (1) as you pass the dumbbells across your body to your right hand (3). Then immediately step forward with the left foot to perform the lunge on the right side. As you lower your hips, bend your right elbow and lift the dumbbells up to shoulder level (4). Pause for 1 count. Lower the dumbbells; lift your hips upward by pressing through the front heel and leg, and step back with your left foot to return to starting position (1). This is 1 repetition.

Repeat 2 to 4 sets of 8 repetitions on the same side. Switch sides and repeat as indicated.

WIDE (PLIÉ) SQUAT WITH UPRIGHT ROW AND OVERHEAD PRESS

Works deltoids, biceps, triceps, middle back, buttocks (gluteals), inner and outer thighs, and quadriceps

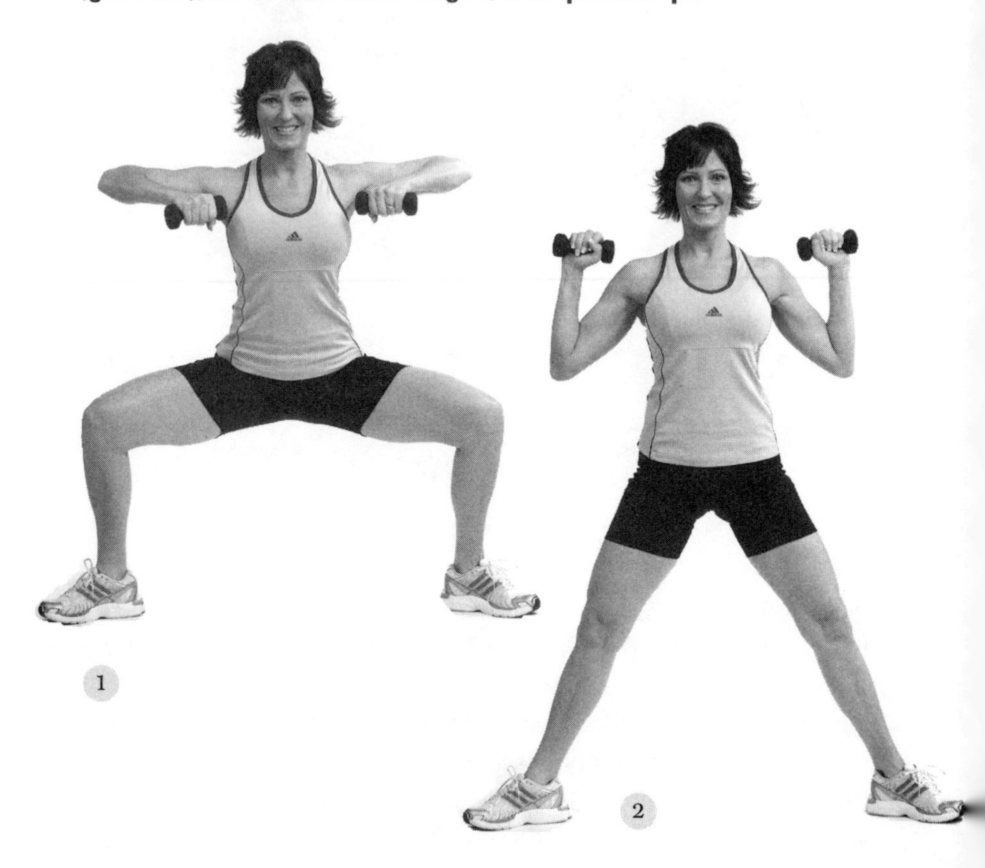

START: Stand with a tall, neutral spine, feet 2 to 3 times wider than hip width apart, and feet and knees turned out comfortably and aligned with each other. Hold the dumbbells together, with palms facing your body and arms narrower than shoulder width. Bend your knees and lower your hips directly down (do not lean forward) into a wide plié squat as you lift your elbows up to shoulder level, until your thighs are parallel with the floor (1).

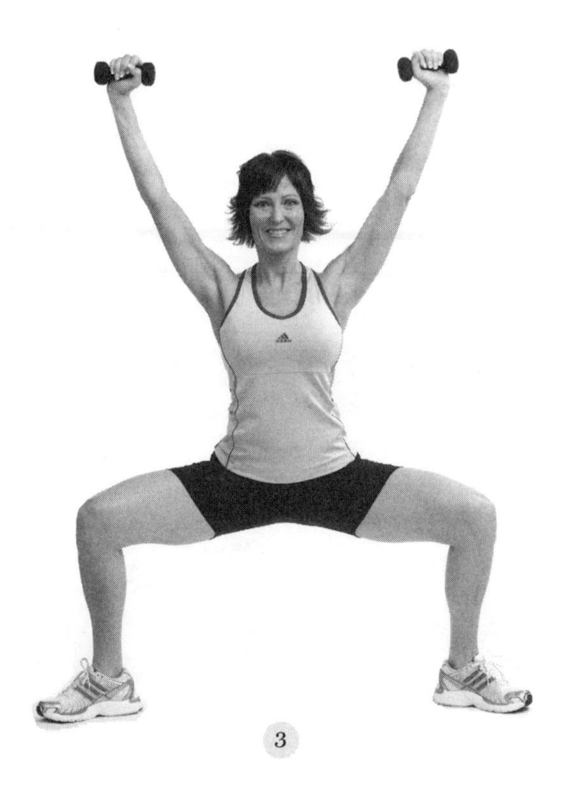

ACTION: Lift the dumbbells up to shoulder level and rise to standing (2) as you pull your elbows down and squeeze your shoulder blades (dumbbells remain at shoulder level); repeat the squat and, as you lower into the squat, press the dumbbells overhead (3). Return to standing as you lower the dumbbells to shoulder level (2), then down in front. This is 1 repetition.

Repeat 2 to 4 sets of 8 to 16 repetitions.

TRICEPS PRESS-UP

Works triceps, pectorals (chest), deltoids (shoulders), and core (abdominals, back, and scapular muscles)

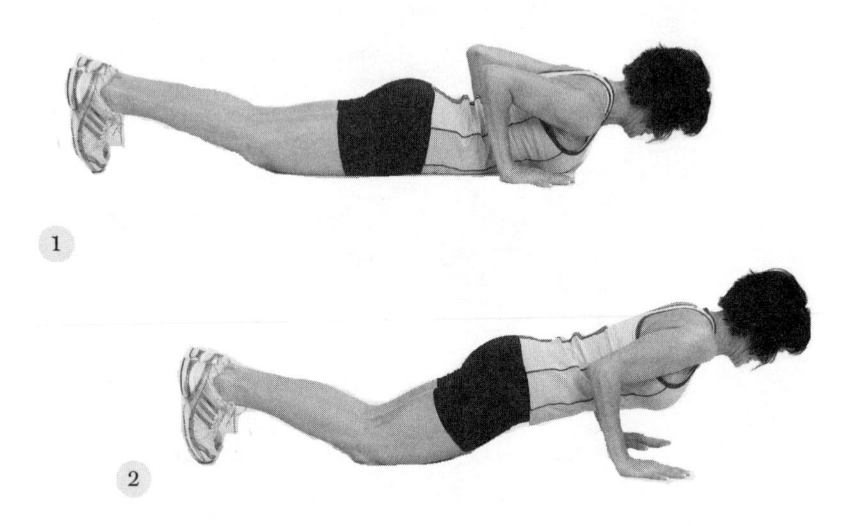

START: Lie face down on the floor or mat, with hands on the floor slightly wider than and below the shoulders, and chin tucked in (eyes focused to the floor). Pull your elbows in close to your rib cage; pull your abdominals up and hold in and squeeze your buttocks (gluteals). Keep them squeezed tight throughout (1).

ACTION: Exhale and push your body halfway up off the floor from your knees to bent-knee plank position (upper arms are parallel with the floor) (2); pause to inhale, then lower slowly toward the floor (rest on the ground only if necessary) and repeat as indicated.

Repeat 2 to 4 sets of 8 to 16 repetitions.

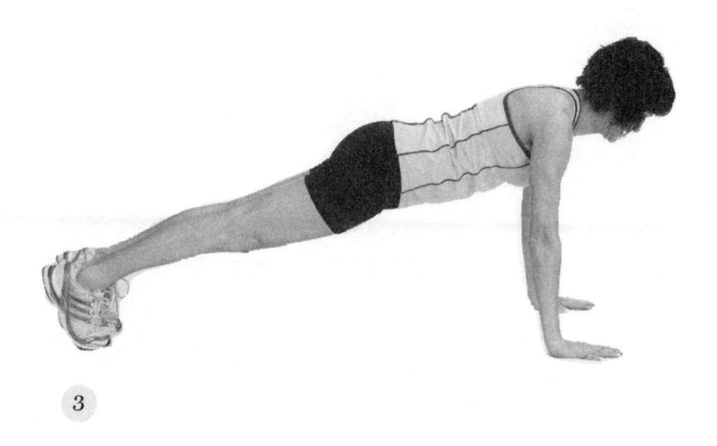

3

PROGRESSION: Push up from your toes until your arms are almost straight; extend your legs straight (3), pause, lower and repeat as indicated.

Repeat 2 sets of 8 repetitions.

Newbody Extra Strength B: Butt, Hips, Back, and Legs

The Extra Strength B routine targets the area that women are most concerned about in terms of their looks and shape. These four whole-body exercises will challenge your strength, balance, coordination, and even your mind because each exercise targets your butt, back, and legs all at once. You will be amazed at how much extra, in terms of results, you will achieve in just 15 minutes.

SIDE LUNGE 'N' LIFT

Works buttocks (gluteals), quadriceps, and hamstrings

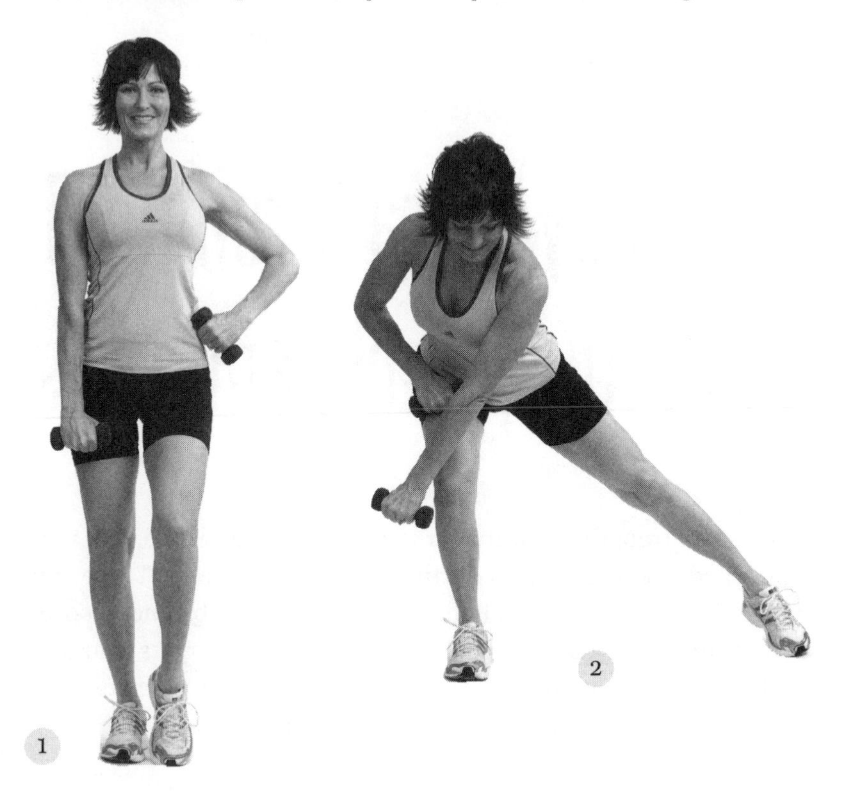

START: Stand with body weight on right leg, left foot in alongside of right foot with heel lifted, and right arm at your side with left hand on your hip. Hold one dumbbell in each hand (1).

ACTION: Step your left leg out to the side and bend your right knee about 45 degrees to lower your hips into a lunge. Lean forward at the hips and reach your left arm across the right knee down toward the floor; squeeze your buttocks to ensure correct alignment of the right knee over the centre of your foot and to maintain your balance (2). Pause for 1 count. Lift hips upwards by pressing up through the right heel and leg, bringing the left leg in to starting position, and repeat as indicated.

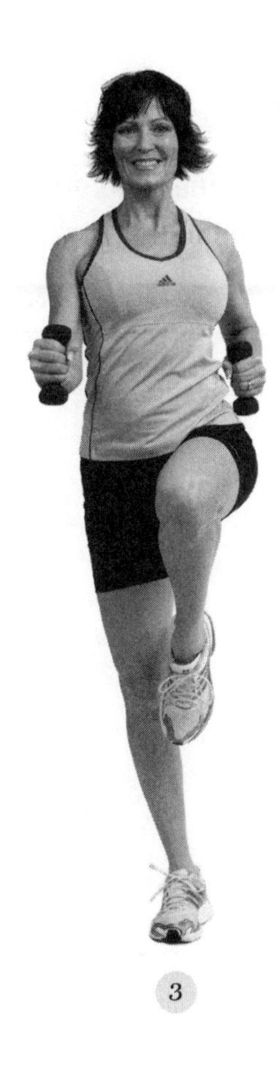

3

Repeat 2 to 4 sets of 8 repetitions. Switch sides and repeat as indicated.

PROGRESSION: Repeat the side lunge as directed and, as you return to starting position, lift your left foot up off floor bending the left knee up to hip level (90 degrees) (3). Pause for 1 count, lower left foot, and repeat as indicated.

Repeat 2 to 4 sets of 8 repetitions.

OPTION: Place both dumbbells in your left hand for a greater challenge or place both hands on the top of the left thigh for greater support.

Repeat 2 to 4 sets of 8 repetitions.

PLIÉ SQUAT WITH LEAN 'N' LIFT

Works buttocks (gluteals), inner and outer thighs, quadriceps, hamstrings, and core (abdominals, back)

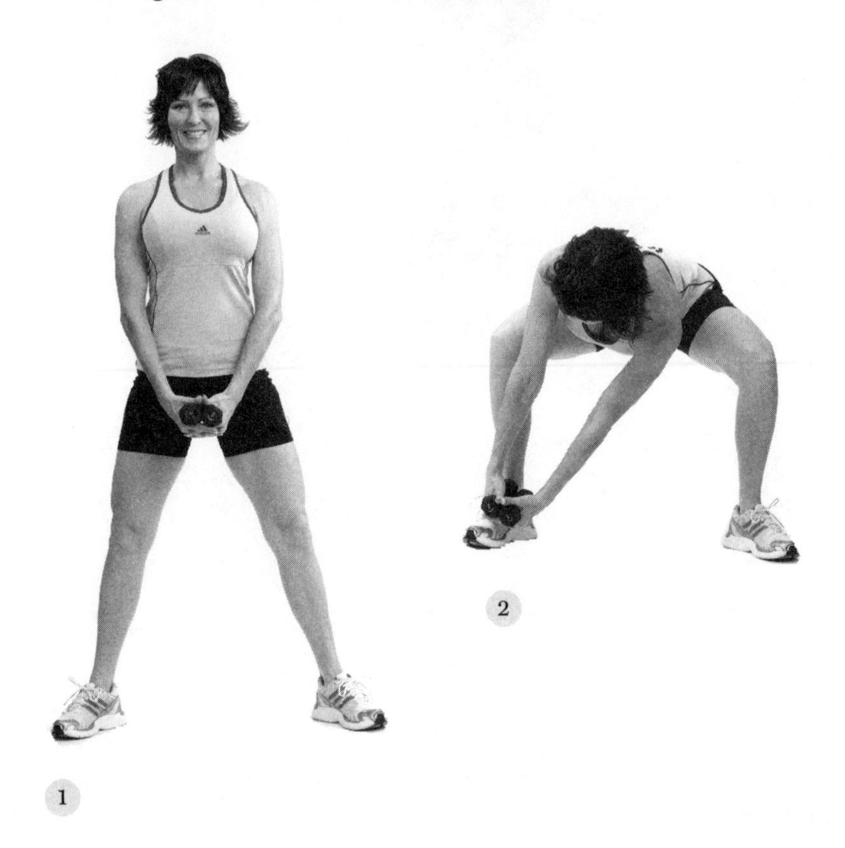

START: Stand with a tall, neutral spine, with feet at least 2 to 3 times wider than your hip width apart, holding dumbbells together with your palms facing each other (bracing together with fingers interlaced). Keep your chest lifted, abdominals pulled in, and buttocks squeezed tight (1).

ACTION: Lean forward from the hips, moving hips back as you lean to lower one or both dumbbells toward the floor and over to the right diagonal (2). Lift with a neutral spine to return to standing;

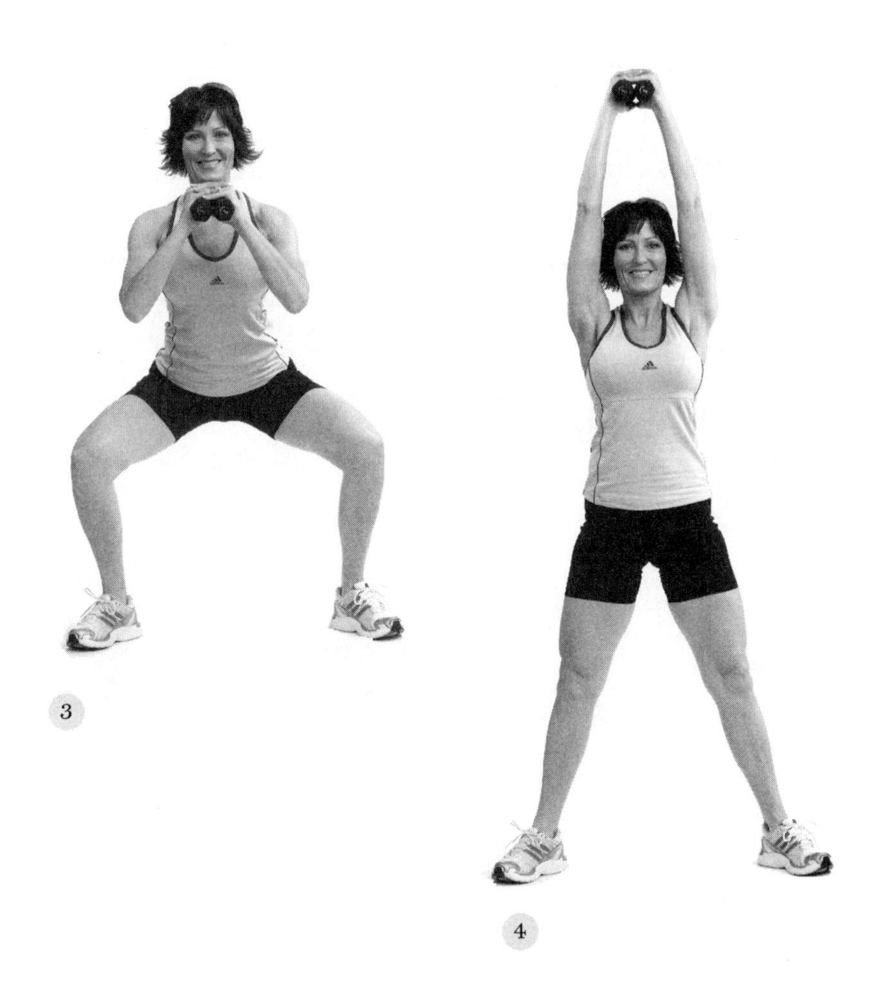

3

4

bend the elbows to lift the dumbbells just above your chest (3), and press the dumbbells overhead (4). Keep bracing the weights together throughout the lean and the lift overhead. Repeat to the left diagonal. This is 1 repetition.

Repeat 2 to 4 sets of 8 repetitions.

OPTION: Repeat the forward lean, lowering the dumbbells down to the diagonal just to the level of the knee for less of a challenge.

MARCHING PLANK

Works buttocks (gluteals), quadriceps, and core (abdominals, back, scapular muscles)

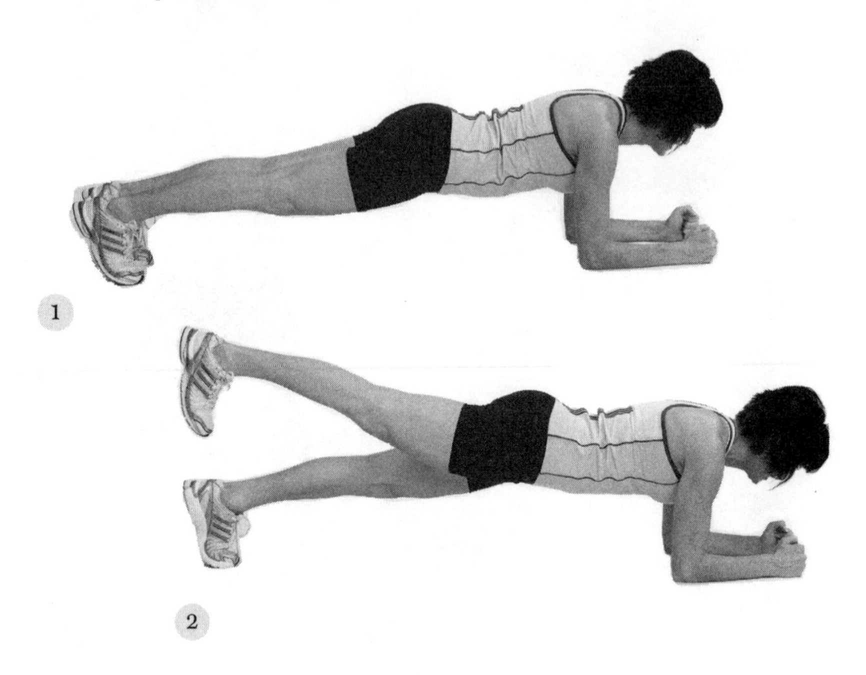

START: Lie face down on the floor, resting on your forearms with palms either together or flat on the ground and elbows directly under your shoulders. Tuck in your chin to keep the neck aligned, pull in your abdominals, and squeeze your buttocks (gluteals). Push off the floor, lifting your hips and knees so that your body is parallel with the ground (1).

ACTION: Keep your head in line with your heels (maintaining a neutral spine) and your hips parallel with the ground by squeezing your shoulder blades together; pull your abdominals in, squeeze your buttocks, and push through your heels. Keep your hips as stable and level as possible as you lift your right leg up just above the level of your hips (2), then switch, alternating in a "marching" action (3). This is 1 repetition.

Repeat 2 to 4 sets of 8 to 16 repetitions.

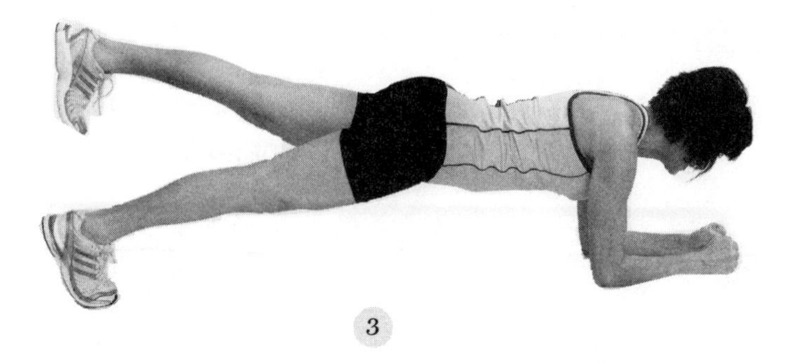

3

PROGRESSION: Repeat the plank (1) as indicated and repeat the "march" out to the side and back in, alternating right and left. This is 1 repetition.

Repeat 2 to 4 sets of 8 to 16 repetitions.

ADVANCED OPTION: Perform the plank from your hands, as opposed to your forearms.

Repeat 2 sets of 8 to 16 repetitions.

SIDE REVOLVING BRIDGE

Works buttocks (gluteals), core (abdominals, back, scapular muscles), and quadratus lumborum (lower back)

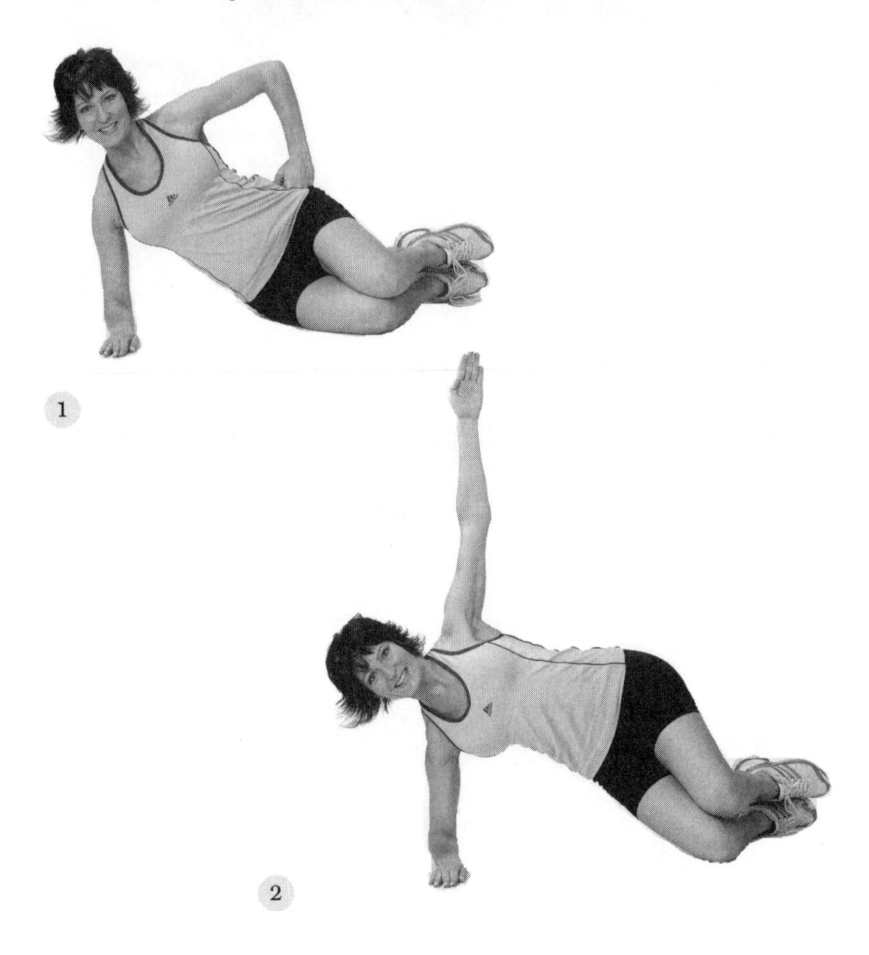

START: Lie on your right side, supporting yourself on your right hip and forearm with your palm flat on the floor. Both knees should be bent (and slightly forward of your hips), and your feet should be behind you. Pull your abdominals in, squeeze your buttocks, press through your forearm, and lift your lower ribs and waist up away from the floor (1).

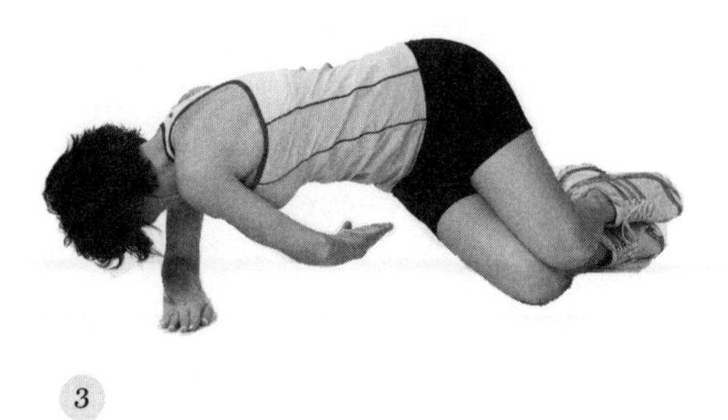

3

ACTION: Lift your hips off the floor, pressing upward through your forearm and lower body, lifting your left arm up toward the ceiling (2). Hold for a count of 5 to 10, then lower. This is 1 repetition.

Repeat 3 to 5 sets of 3 repetitions on each side.

PROGRESSION: Repeat the side bridge as indicated (2); reach down and under your ribs toward your bottom hip with your left hand and hold for one count (3); return hand to (2) and repeat 4 to 8 repetitions. Return to starting position (1) and switch sides.

Repeat 2 sets of 4 to 8 repetitions on each side.

Newbody Extra Strength C: Core Abdominals, Hips, Back, and Shoulders

The Extra Strength C routine targets the core, or "control centre," of your body—where all movement begins. The muscles that surround the shoulder girdle, the spine, and the hips together are referred to as the core muscles, and it is the core muscles that are responsible for the way we sit, stand, and move around. The majority of back pain or poor posture comes from having a weak core, so that is why these four extra strength exercises that make up the C routine are programmed into your Newbody Workout Schedule three times a week.

STANDING STAR SEQUENCE

Works buttocks (gluteals), core (abdominals, back, and scapular muscles), quadratus lumborum (lower back), and erector spinals

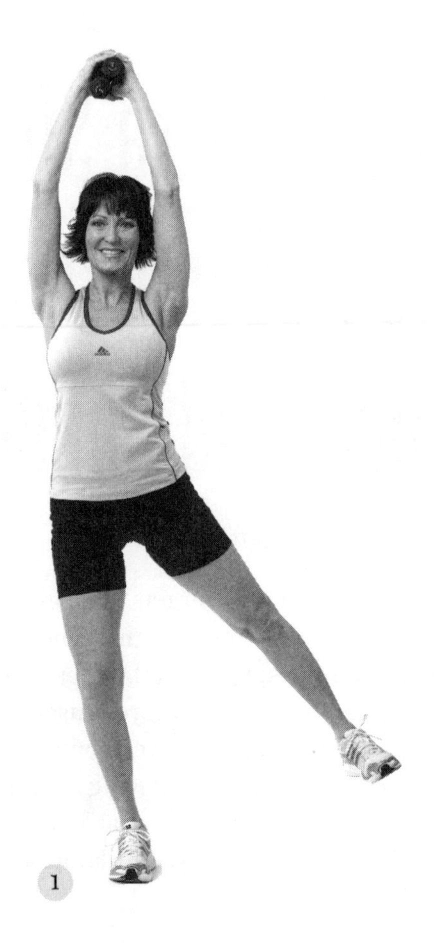

START: Stand in a tall, neutral position with feet hip width apart and arms at sides. Transfer body weight onto your right foot and lift your left foot off the floor. Lift both arms overhead, holding one or both dumbbells (1). Pull your shoulders down away from your ears, pull in your abdominals, squeeze your buttocks, and band your right knee to help maintain your balance.

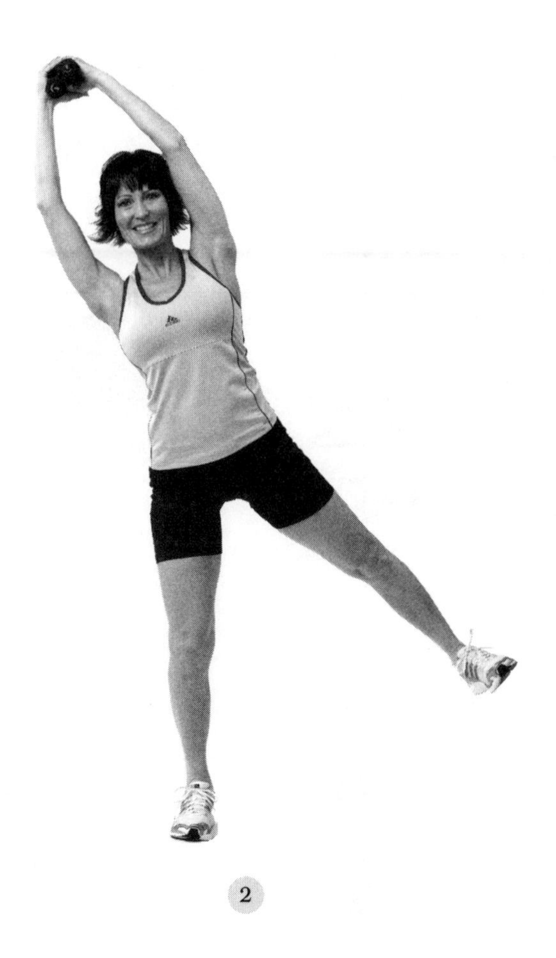

2

ACTION: Lift your left foot higher as you lean over toward the right side (2). Hold for 5 to 10 counts, then return to starting position. This is 1 repetition. Repeat as indicated.

Repeat 3 sets of 5 repetitions to each side.

ABDOMINAL CRUNCH WITH HEEL DROP

Works the abdominals

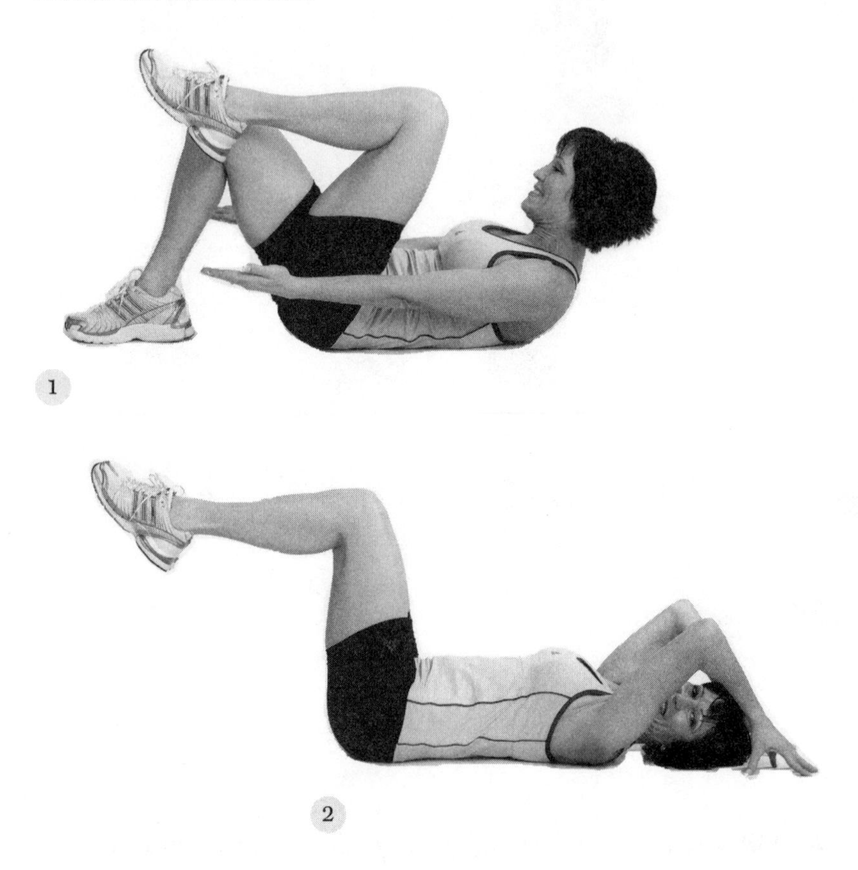

START: Lie on the ground or a mat with knees bent and feet on the ground. Place hands alongside your torso with palms facing up.

ACTION: Pull your abdominals in toward your spine as you draw your chin in to help lift your upper torso off the floor, moving your rib cage toward your hips while at the same time lifting your left foot off the floor and pulling your knee toward your chest. Exhale as you lift, hold for 1 count to inhale (1), then lower your left foot and repeat with the right leg. This is 1 repetition.

Repeat 2 to 4 sets of 8 to 16 repetitions.

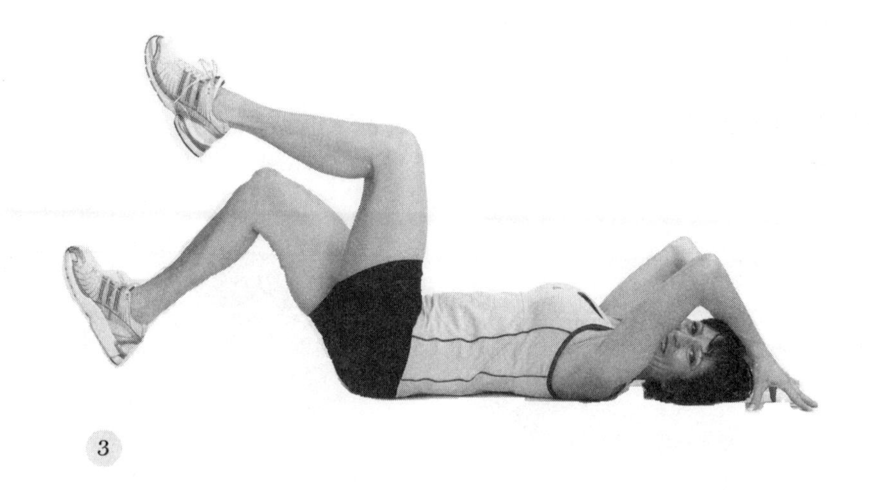

3

PROGRESSION: Lift your arms overhead with elbows bent at 90 degrees and fingers touching the floor; bring both feet up off the floor with knees directly over the hips to start (2). Exhale and lower your right heel toward the ground, without any motion through your core (do not allow your lower back to lift) (3). Hold for 1 count; inhale, and return to starting position to repeat with the left side. This is 1 repetition.

ADVANCED OPTION: Extend the right leg straight out as you lower it toward the floor, hold for 1 count, inhale, return to starting position (2), and repeat to the other side. This is 1 repetition.

Repeat 2 to 4 sets of 8 to 16 repetitions.

ROTATING PLANK

Works core (abdominals, back, and scapular muscles), buttocks (gluteals), and shoulders

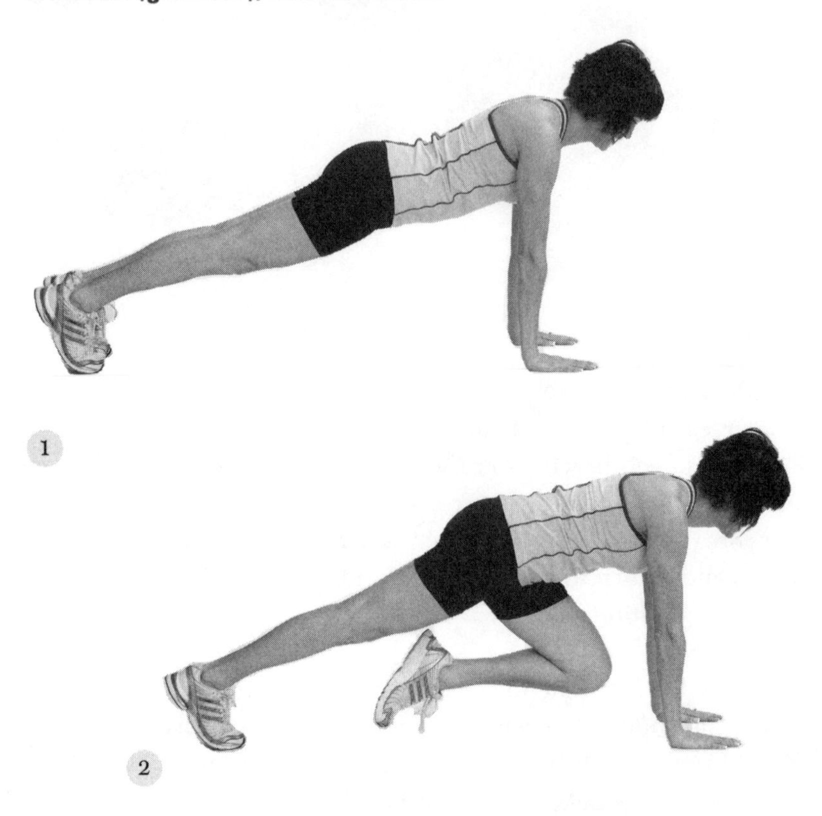

START: Kneel on all fours with hands just wider than shoulder width apart and elbows slightly bent and in line with wrists, fingers facing forward. Tuck in your chin to keep the neck aligned, pull in abdominal muscles, and squeeze your buttocks as you extend your legs out behind you one at a time. Support your weight on your hands and toes (1). Lift your left foot off the floor and bring your knee toward your chest (2). Hold for 1 count, and exhale. Inhale as you return to starting position (1) and repeat with the right leg for 1 repetition.

Repeat 2 sets of 4 to 8 repetitions.

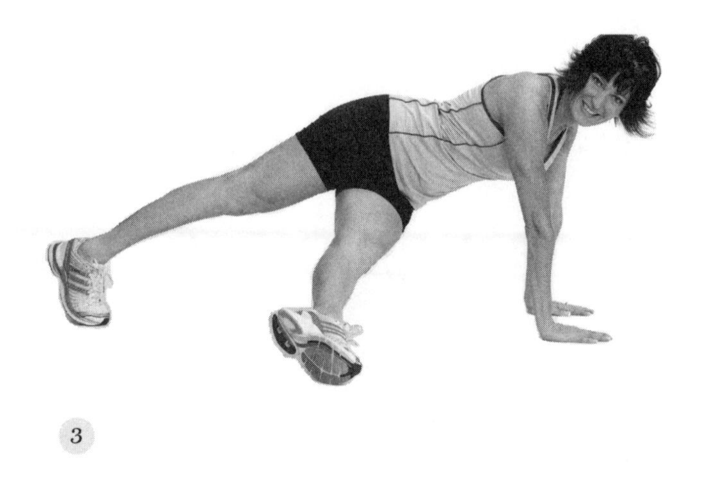

3

PROGRESSION: Repeat as indicated with the left (1), (2); then bring your left knee toward your right and extend at the knee to straighten the leg. Hold for 1 count and exhale (3). As you inhale, bend the knee and return to starting position and repeat with the right. This is 1 repetition.

Repeat 2 sets of 4 to 8 repetitions.

V-SIT WITH ROTATION

Works core (abdominals, back, and scapular muscles) and erector spinals

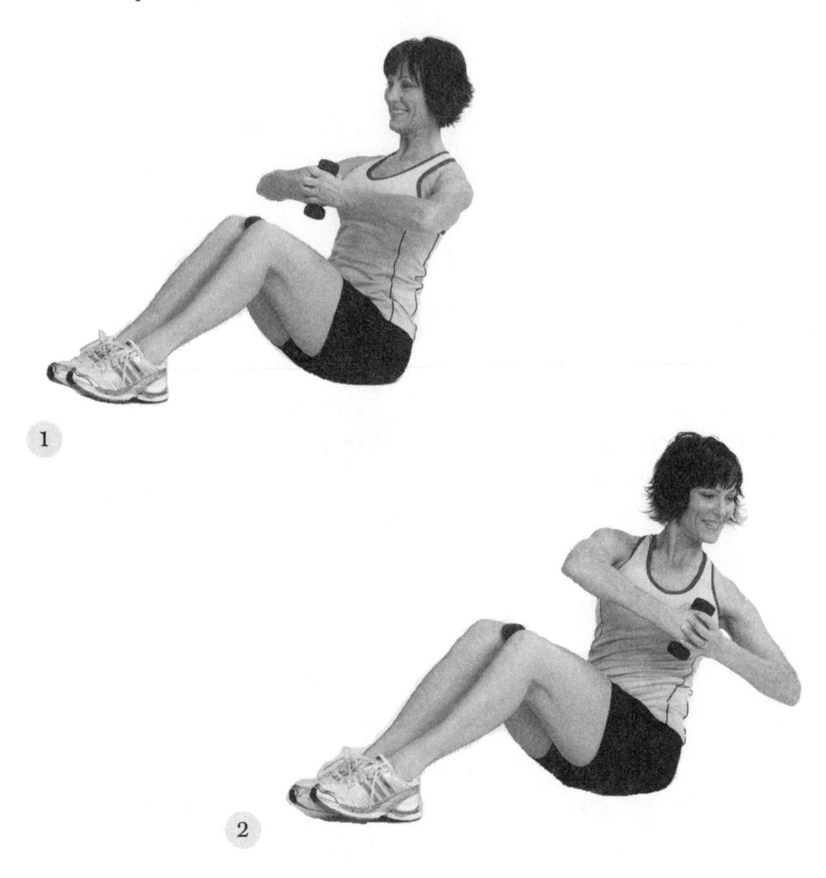

START: Sit on the floor or a mat with both knees bent at 90 degrees and feet on the ground. Place one dumbbell between your knees and squeeze to help stabilize your lower body and core. Lift chest up, keeping your chin level with the floor to maintain a neutral spine. Bend your elbows; interlace your fingers, or hold on to one dumbbell just below the chest with your elbows lifted out to the side (1).

ACTION: Anchor your heels down onto the floor by pressing down. As you exhale, rotate your torso left, bringing your left elbow toward the ground and right elbow across to the left. Hold for 1 count (2), inhale, and return to centre; rotate to the other side. This is 1 repetition.

Repeat 2 to 4 sets of 8 to 16 repetitions.

PROGRESSION: Repeat the V-sit, rotating to the left with your elbows as you lift the left foot off the floor. Hold for 1 count, inhale, and return to centre; repeat to the other side, lifting your right foot. This is 1 repetition.

Repeat 2 to 4 sets of 8 to 16 repetitions.

3

Newbody Mind

Exercising makes me feel good all over, and while I love the physical aspects and the payoffs I see in the mirror, I know that the effects that exercising has on my mind will keep me coming back too! During a vigorous workout (whether I am leading a Newbody class, lifting weights, or running), I feel fantastic—and that is often the result of feel-good chemicals called endorphins that are released in the brain during strenuous exercise. After a Newbody class, I feel energized yet calmer and more relaxed, and I think that has to do with the fact that I've burned up or worked out some of the bad stress I've been accumulating. The point is that exercise is good for your body *and* your mind, whether you're doing specific mind–body exercises or are exercising indiscriminately!

The mind–body connection has increasingly been in the spotlight during the last few decades, and health experts and scientists know a whole lot more about it than they did before. In a nutshell, your body reacts in physiological ways to the way you think, feel, and act. For example, when you're chronically stressed or upset, you may develop high blood pressure or depression. (Are these things related? Many health experts would say yes.) On the other hand, when you de-stress your body regularly through exercise and other stress-management techniques, you tend to feel calmer overall and you can usually better handle a situation when it does get out of hand (such as getting stuck in traffic or losing your keys). Many experts also suggest that reducing chronic stress supports better health overall. The health benefits range from losing weight to sleeping more restfully and strengthening immunity against illness!

Mind-body exercise taps into these principles. Exercises such as yoga, Tai Chi, and Qigong combine body movement with mental focus and controlled breathing to improve strength, balance, coordination, flexibility, and overall health. But other exercise helps too: I always tell my Newbody participants that since they brought their mind to class, they may as well exercise it too—and we do! The cross-crawl exercise is one of the aspects of mind fitness that I incorporate into the Newbody workout. Cross-crawl is a brain exercise that improves mind-body coordination—where you reach the right hand across the body to the left hip, knee, and/or foot as you lift it, then do the same thing for the left hand to the right side of your body, and repeat in an alternating manner—as if you were marching. While this exercise is about training basic motor skills, it also helps coordinate the right and left sides of the brain by exercising the information flow between the two hemispheres. And that's useful for spelling, writing, listening, reading, and comprehension!

At the same time, any activity that takes your mind off all the stressors of life (the worry about getting a report done or whether you'll get a bank loan) is a form of mind-body exercise too. For example, a sport or recreational activity that requires technical skills—such as downhill skiing, playing golf or tennis, or lifting weights—is a form of mind-body exercise because you can't think of much outside of the sport or physical activity when you're doing it (you're focused on getting down the hill in one piece or hitting the ball). In that way, focusing your mind on accomplishing skills such as these helps to relieve symptoms associated with excessive stress, such as anxiety, fatigue, high blood pressure, and so on. It's wonderful and very therapeutic.

The Newbody program encapsulates this principle too. The aerobic and strength-training portions in general help tackle all your stressors: while you're doing the program, you're burning calories and battling all those stress bunnies that hop around in your brain! The highly repetitious, easy-to-follow exercise sequences require your concentration as well as your coordination—and that means you're focused on achieving a goal and therefore can't dwell on any worries. I am always amazed that the worries or problems that sat on my mind going into a class seem much smaller or have left my mind by the time I have finished my workout.

Experts recommend that you challenge and condition all your muscles *and* your mind at every stage of your life—and Newbody fits the bill every step of the way. Of course there are lots of other ways to challenge and condition your mind and body—including line dancing and chess, or learning to sculpt or paint. I started ballroom dancing a few years ago with my husband. All these learning situations combine thinking and doing, and they're as important as moving your body physically on a daily basis.

There's also a growing body of scientific research that shows how important physical exercise is for your mind power—if you don't use it, you lose it! For example, if your biggest complaint as you get older is a foggy memory, lace up your fitness shoes. Researchers have found that the more people exercise, the less cognitive decline they see, particularly in women—cognitive decline is those annoying memory lapses and problems with reasoning and learning. People who exercise have a better memory. Furthermore, it doesn't matter how old you are or how active you have been throughout your life. Regular exercise may even help reverse this type of cognitive decline. Regular exercisers are less likely to develop memory loss and confusion (often diagnosed as dementia or Alzheimer's). They're happier too—research has shown that aerobic exercise can be just as effective as medication in decreasing depression.

How much exercise are we talking about? That's the best part of all: only a minimum of 30 minutes at least twice a week!

NEWBODY TIP: As you focus your mind on the specific muscle and/or movement, you are actually learning and/or rehearsing skills as they relate to daily living and increasing muscle recruitment. Both these benefits will lead to improvement in performance both in terms of improving fitness level and functional ability. Consider how much more confident and able you will be to push yourself up off the floor and protect yourself from injury if you fall when you train your body with push-ups. This is why all women should include push-ups in their fitness program.

FEED YOUR MIND—AND YOUR MOOD

- **GLUCOSE** (sugar) is the brain's primary source of energy. When you eat carbohydrates (such as breads, pasta, and wholegrain cereal), they are converted to glucose by the body. When you don't eat carbohydrates, you're essentially starving your brain—and it's no wonder you can't think clearly and get cranky. Also, eating carbohydrates triggers the release of an amino acid (tryptophan, which is converted to serotonin) that boosts your mood and may help reduce pain, decrease appetite, and produce a sense of calm. It's interesting to note that dieters who cut out carbohydrates tend to become depressed about two weeks into their diet, which is about the time their serotonin levels have dropped due to decreased carbohydrate intake. (One serving of a carbohydrate at each meal is a good idea whether you're eating to lose weight or eating for good health.)

- **PROTEIN** provides the building blocks for the brain and allows your brain cells to communicate with one another. So eating lean sources of protein at every meal (meat, fish, poultry, low fat yoghurt, cheese or milk, soy, beans, lentils) affects your alertness and ability to think clearly throughout the day.

- **MICRONUTRIENTS**, such as all the wonderful vitamins and minerals in fruits and vegetables, and those in a supplement form, are important for the overall growth and functioning of the brain, so aim for one of each at every meal.

- **FATS**, the good kind such as omega-3 fatty acids, are what the brain uses to create cells that allow you to think (the brain is more than 60 percent fat). Omega-3 fats are found in oily fish such as salmon, tuna, cod, sardines and herring—choose 3 servings per week. A heaping tablespoon of grounds seeds each day (flaxseeds, sesame, sunflower, hemp, and pumpkin seeds) sprinkled on or in your foods energizes your meals and your mind.

- **WATER** keeps your brain hydrated and helps it to metabolize food and carry out chemical reactions in the body. The rule of thumb: eight 8-ounce (250 mL) glasses of water a day. You can count any (decaffeinated) liquid as water, and remember, many fruits and vegetables are comprised mostly of liquid. Drink more water when you're exercising or under a lot of stress—these are times when we sweat a lot and increase the risk of dehydration, which can affect alertness and concentration too.

Willpower

Research has found that willpower is a mental muscle—and there are ways to strengthen your willpower.

- **FOOD.** Remember, glucose fuels the brain so if the brain is running on empty, it's going to be in a vulnerable position. Having a bite to eat will boost willpower. Dieters who eat several small meals a day appear to do better at sticking to a diet than dieters who skip meals. (They also do better at keeping to a fitness program because they have the energy.)

- **VISUALIZATION.** If you need a bit of willpower to do your Newbody workout today, visualize yourself in a bikini next summer ... that should help get you there. If you need a bit of willpower to do your Newbody workout today, revisit your "dream" goal and the emotions that go with it. Visualize yourself having achieved the goal ... now you just need to go and do it.

HOW EXERCISE AFFECTS YOUR MIND

- Aerobic exercise generally helps regulate the nervous system and reduces stress. It increases blood flow to your brain and helps to calm your mind. All the systemic changes that occur (stronger heart and lungs, stronger bones, better blood and oxygen delivery) add up to less fatigue and more focus and energy all day.

- When you strength train muscles, something wonderful happens inside your head. But it's not magic: it's physiological and psychological—you feel stronger, inside and out. Studies have shown time and again that strength training improves self-esteem in many women. Even a modest regimen—working out with weights for 20 to 30 minutes, 2 to 3 times a week—can improve how you feel about your physical abilities and therefore improve your overall self-concept. Think about it. When you strength train, you can lose weight, build beautiful, toned muscles, and not only look fabulous at any age but feel more confident and empowered.

- Relaxation training—meditation, yoga, and Tai Chi, or simply focusing on your breathing for 1 to 10 minutes at a time—decreases muscle tension, lowers blood pressure, slows down heart rate and breathing, and reduces stress hormones, which allows you to think more clearly and feel calm and happy.

- When I need to clear my mind, I often take a walk around the block. I always come back refreshed because physical movement increases breathing and heart rate, which increases blood and oxygen circulation in the brain—just what you need when you feel foggy and overwhelmed by too many thoughts in your head. Health Canada recommends at least 30 minutes of physical activity every day. Take a 10-minute walk around the block right now—to clear your mind and start building toward that 30-minute goal. Chunking up activities in 10-minute blocks is as effective for improving your overall health as completing your 30 minutes all at once.

- Help wake up your brain in the morning by thinking positive thoughts while you're still lying in bed and by consciously wiggling your fingers and toes several times in any way that feels good. This is a good revitalization and centring technique that also helps to mobilize the joints and activate the nerves that stimulate your mind and internal organs.

NEWBODY TIP: Motivate your mind and body with music. Music is a terrific motivator during exercise, and listening to upbeat music (at a moderate speed) while doing the Newbody exercises will help improve your rhythm and keep you energized for the entire 30 minutes. Listening to music can also ease symptoms of depression

Q&A *with* Mo

Q My memory is not as good as it used to be. Is this aging or is it menopause?

A The North American Menopause Society says there is no firm evidence that memory or other cognitive skills actually decline because of natural menopause. However, that's not to say that difficulty remembering and concentrating during perimenopause and the years right after menopause doesn't happen. What we do know for sure is that getting enough sleep is important for having a clear mind and memory every day. But also being physically and mentally active may help prevent memory loss. Just as you train your heart and other muscles, it's important to exercise your mind. Programs such as Newbody provide the right kind of training—you have to concentrate to follow the exercise progressions and you mimic movements of everyday life (for example, reaching across the body to pick something up) and challenge your body and mind to work effectively together. And this takes us right back to the place where it all begins—the control room: the brain.

associated with stress. Listening to your favourite tunes will reduce cortisol levels, high blood pressure, and fatigue, and boost your mood.

EXERCISE ALWAYS HAS A PLACE IN YOUR LIFE

Learning how to juggle all the demands in our lives isn't easy, and working moms especially often have to cope with their family's needs, the demands of their jobs, and then if there's any time left over, maybe their own needs. Unfortunately, it's really easy to talk yourself into quitting exercise, especially when you're chronically overloaded with stressors. But honestly, stressful times are the times when a woman needs regular exercise most, as exercise provides a great escape from all the demands in your life and is a great way to give yourself some well-deserved tender loving care. Exercise is never something you should cross off your to-do list. It's one of the easiest ways to feel good about yourself, have more energy, and feel in control of your body and calm in your mind. The bottom line: if you don't take care of yourself, beginning with your own health, you will be less able to take care of others.

4

Newbody Shoulders and Arms

SHOULDERS

"Stand up straight and pull your shoulders back, Mo!"

I must have heard that a million times when I was growing up. But you know something? My mother's constant reminders paid off. I grew up with a keen interest and eye for how we stand and should move, and I ended up in careers that have been all about the body. First, I studied to become a physiotherapist and learned the musculoskeletal and other systems of the body. Today, I am still super-aware of my posture, especially when I am teaching Newbody and other exercise classes. (I like to think of myself as the posture police!) But there are still some days when I catch myself or get caught slouching—at my computer, on an airplane, or while standing in a lineup.

Of course, good posture isn't just about your shoulders. It's about your whole body and mind—and your posture says a lot about you. Think about it: when you want to imitate someone who is sad or depressed, all you have to do is slump your shoulders forward, round your back, and look down at the floor. Research has proven that this type of body language is often a reflection of the way a person feels about herself. Someone who has poor posture not only lacks strength and body awareness but may also lack self-esteem, self-confidence, or energy.

On the other hand, a properly aligned body—which is when the chin is tucked in (retracted) and the neck and spine are elongated, the shoulders are back and relaxed down, the chest is open, and the head is up—has energy and looks healthy and strong. And when you look healthy and strong, you feel good too. Research concurs. Studies have shown there is a correlation between physical strength in the upper body and improved self-efficacy that can be up to 70 percent!

Good posture is healthier too. When your body is properly aligned, it is well balanced, with minimum stress and strain on supporting structures such as the vertebral joints of the spine, spinal nerves, muscles, ligaments, and connective tissues. Good posture also supports proper functioning of the internal organs—for example, the lungs have the space they need for full expansion and you breathe easier.

For strong and shapely shoulders, the Newbody program incorporates exercises that target the muscles that support and define the shoulders, and I always include reminders about being in proper position and posture for the exercise in my descriptions. To strengthen the major muscles of the shoulders, I've included different types of overhead presses. Front, side, and rear arm raises and a variety of rowing exercises target each part of the shoulder as well as the upper back and arms. A combination of all these movements also works the rotator cuff (the group of muscles that surround and support the shoulder joint). We always balance the exercises we do too, so every push or press is balanced with a pull or row. However, you may notice that you perform more repetitions focused on pulling and lifting than pushing and lowering—this helps to offset natural muscle imbalances in the shoulder, upper back, and chest region.

All this work will pay off with new shapely shoulders—which some people think are a woman's sexiest body part!

Keep your shoulders strong for life

Did you know that the shoulder has the widest range of motion of any joint in the body? Its flexibility lets you do everything from taking a powerful slapshot on the hockey rink, to moving the stove so you can clean behind it, to throwing a ball as far as you can for your dog, or doing a push-up. But the structure of this joint also makes the shoulder vulnerable to injury. The boniness of the shoulder makes it unstable. Since a number of muscles go across the shoulder joint, they are all subject to pinching and even tearing over time. Age, strain, and overuse, combined with the shoulder's structure, can lead to injuries. Here are ways to prevent shoulder injury:

- Power up your posture! Tight chest muscles and rounded shoulders caused by prolonged sitting at your desk or in front of the computer terminal or television ends up restricting your arm movement and strength. When your shoulders are misaligned, even simple arms movements that involve your shoulder can cause injury. The solution: strengthen your shoulder-blade muscles with exercises and practise good posture when you stand and sit.
- Strength and stability exercises for the shoulders can help. Strength training with free weights is great.
- Exercise for strong and supple shoulders includes swimming, yoga, Pilates, stretching (flexibility training), and rowing.
- Weight-bearing exercise for the upper body, such as push-ups and planks (just like low-impact exercise for the lower body), overloads your muscles and bones to build strength and resilience.
- A high-calcium, high-fibre, low-fat diet in general is good for bones. Good sources of calcium include dairy products, fish with bones, green leafy vegetables, almonds, seeds, beans and soy, and fortified cereals.

Age-related loss of strength, muscle mass, and bone density, especially in women, can be lessened by strengthening exercises. And it's better late than never. Studies have shown that seniors who strength train consistently for 6 weeks in a row or longer can improve their muscular strength, bone density, balance, aerobic capacity, flexibility, and energy. They end up being more independent and self-confident, at lower risk for falls, and more positive in outlook too.

The key is overloading muscle to prevent loss of muscle mass and strength. Start a strength-training program such as Newbody and be sure to see your doctor first if you haven't exercised for a while.

De-stress your neck and shoulders

Our lives are full of ways to strain the neck and shoulders—for example, leaning forward to read small print on your computer or holding your shoulders stiffly while you're concentrating on work. Here are some ways to relieve some of the strain:

- **NECK.** Use the tips of your thumbs to work circles into the taut muscles at the sides of your neck. Change to your fingertips and use lighter pressure working down the sides from behind your ears toward your shoulders.

- **SHOULDERS.** Reach one arm across the front of your body and press your fingers firmly into muscles above the opposite shoulder blade for 10 to 20 seconds. Switch sides.

- **FOR BOTH.** Raise the top of your shoulders up to your ears while breathing in through your nose. Relax and lower shoulders as far down as possible as you exhale.

ARMS

Whether you're wearing a tank top, a swimsuit, or a sleeveless dress, there's nothing more beautiful than toned arms and sculpted shoulders—and the best way to get this look is by strength training regularly. The secret to getting the arms you've always desired is to lift enough weight, including your own body weight, so you're adequately overloading your arms and shoulders. The good news is that it will be easier than you think, and if you've got concerns about bulking up, put them aside. Unlike men, women don't produce the testosterone necessary to create big and bulky muscles. Plus, you would have to lift extremely heavy weights—and with my Newbody workout and Extra Strength A routine, you use very light weights and high repetitions. I am certain that you want a proportionate, toned, and balanced physique, and to accomplish that, you must build up your upper body. I've designed the Newbody exercises to target arm muscles (the biceps and triceps) and the naturally weaker muscles that surround the shoulders, chest, and upper back, at the same time—and this is perfect for a woman's

Q&A *with* Mo

Q My computer whiz daughter is only 12 years old and she has the posture of an old woman ... rounded shoulders and hunched upper back with a poking chin. Will her posture be like that for life?

A If nothing changes, then nothing changes, but if you jump on your daughter's posture now you will be able to correct it. She's not alone. Many young people who spend a lot of time in front of a computer monitor are showing signs that the muscles that support the neck and upper back, shoulders, and spine are weak while the muscles of the front of the shoulders and chest (including the abdominals and hip flexors) are tight. It is highly likely your daughter's poor posture is affecting the way she walks and negatively affecting her general disposition and mood. Encourage her to get active at least 30 minutes every day. Suggest or provide your daughter with fun opportunities (after-school team sports, neighbourhood play groups, swimming or dancing lessons) to learn activity and address these muscle imbalances too. Getting active after school or before or right after dinner will help limit the amount of time she is sitting in front of the computer or television where poor posture develops. You might also provide your daughter with a personal trainer or the opportunity to exercise with you and within 6 weeks you and your daughter will see a visible improvement in her posture. It might be fun to exercise together.

body and muscular structure. By developing strength and shape in your arms, you will be able to increase your physical capabilities for doing all the things you need to do in daily life, from lifting heavy bags of groceries or your suitcase to holding and hugging your kids.

YOUR MUSCLES

Beginning around age 40, adults lose up to 5 percent of muscle mass every decade. That decline increases to 1 to 2 percent a year after age 50. This downhill decline in muscle tissue equates to a significant amount of strength loss—up to 50 percent between the ages of 40 and 60. Women can't spare this amount of strength because there's not a lot of strength in the upper body, relative to the lower body, to begin with. The bad news is that as you lose strength, you lose function and even bone density.

We need muscle and we need to be strong so we can remain independent. The more muscle we have on our bodies, especially our chest, back, shoulders, and arms, the more self-reliant we will be as we get older.

The good news is that muscle mass will increase at any age in response to exercise. Scientific research has shown that strength training performed 2 to 3 times a week using a moderate amount of resistance will improve strength and function in young and old alike.

Building strong upper bodies makes you stronger in other ways too. Research has shown that when older women particularly participate in strength-training programs, their self-confidence and self-esteem improve. Of course, these improvements also have an effect on quality of life!

Strength training also plays a role in weight control. Someone who has a lot of muscle on their body has a higher metabolic rate compared to someone who has a lot of fat on their body. A higher metabolic rate burns more calories even at rest. That's because muscle consumes calories while stored fat uses very little energy.

YOUR BONES

Strengthening muscles and bones is an important way to protect yourself from injuries if you fall. When a person falls, the immediate reaction and first line of defence is to reach out and break the fall with the arms. You often hear about women who have broken a wrist or upper arm, or dislocated their shoulder, as a result of breaking a fall. But regular exercise to strengthen bones and muscles will keep you in the best possible position. Physical activity of any kind puts an increased "load" or force on bones—and they respond by forming new bone and remodelling the bone to be stronger. At the same time, exercising to strengthen muscles also strengthens the bones that they're attached to. An interesting study showed that professional tennis players' bones in the arm that holds the racquet are much larger and stronger than the bones in the other arm. It's another case of "use it or lose it."

FIVE REASONS TO PICK UP FREE WEIGHTS

1. Free weights require more balance and coordination and recruitment of more muscles, especially the deeper, smaller stabilizer muscles. If you're doing a standing dumbbell shoulder press overhead, you work the deltoid muscle of the shoulder, the triceps in the upper arms, the upper and lower back, abdominals, and gluteals at the hip just to maintain your balance and position. Even your leg muscles have to get involved to help you lift the weight overhead. All these muscles are completely engaged as you lift, balance, and return to your starting position. Of course, the heavier the load being pushed or pressed overhead, the more muscle work involved. All this adds up to more calories burned.

2. Free weights allow greater range of motion and exercise variation.

3. The use of free weights develops "functional strength"—the type of strength and "transfer effect" that will make performing activities of daily living so much easier and efficient. Being able to lift stacks of dishes up into or out of a cupboard without help is self-empowering, especially as you get older. For women, being able to pull your body up to a chin-up bar is also empowering. (Try it: you'll see.)

4. Free weights are inexpensive and non-intimidating.

5. Free weights are portable, take up little space, and can be used at home or when travelling.

NEWBODY TIP: There are 3500 calories in 1 pound of fat weight. The number of calories burned in a 30-minute aerobic workout is between 220 and 400 calories (depending on intensity and size of individual). If you move your arms as vigorously as you move your lower body in aerobic activities such as walking, running, or swimming, you can increase caloric expenditure by as much as 35 percent. Imagine what you will accomplish with light hand-weights (dumbbells) in tow during your 30-minute Newbody workout!

PUSH-UPS: ARMED FOR ACTION

Push-ups are one of the best exercises you can do:

- Push-ups build bone and muscle strength in your arms, shoulder girdle, and upper spine.
- They functionally mimic movements that we make in daily life, such as pushing ourselves up off the floor or protecting ourselves from a fall by reaching out with one hand to brace ourselves and break the fall.
- They create lean muscle mass that raises your metabolism—so you burn more calories.
- Push-ups work all the muscles in your arms (biceps, triceps, and forearms).
- They strengthen and tone your shoulders too (strong shoulders and arms help you safely lift heavier weight).
- Push-ups work the chest (for a perky chest and breasts).
- Push-ups build up the muscles in your upper back (these muscles carry the entire body). And stronger back muscles also help power up posture and lower the risk for back injury.
- You don't need any equipment—you use your own body for resistance.

There are lots of fun and different ways to do a push-up. Here are my favourites:

- **BASIC PUSH-UP.** Lie face down on the floor or mat with hands on the floor, placed wider than and just below the shoulders, and chin tucked in (eyes looking to the floor). Your legs are straight and slightly apart (feet are hip width with toes tucked under). Pull your abdominals up and in, squeeze your buttocks (gluteals) and hold throughout. Exhale and push your body up off the floor from your knees to a bent-knee, push-up position or from your toes for a greater challenge. Pause to inhale, then slowly lower halfway to the floor. Pause to inhale. Repeat 2 to 3 sets of 5 to 15 repetitions.

- **WALL PUSH-UP.** Stand about 3 feet in front of the wall, arms extended, palms pressing against the wall (placed wider than and just below shoulder level). Lean your body toward the wall, keeping it straight, abdominals pulled in, and buttocks tight. Pause to inhale. Exhale and push your body back with your arms until you are once again in a standing position. Repeat 2 to 3 sets of 10 to 15 repetitions.

- **NARROW AND WIDE GRIP PUSH-UP.** This is your basic push-up but with varying widths of hand positions. For the narrow grip position, place your hands on the floor just below your shoulders and slightly wider than shoulder width. Keep elbows in close alongside your rib cage as you perform the basic push-up (targets the arms). For the wide grip position, perform the same exercise, but place your hands on the floor at twice the width of your shoulders (targets the chest).

Q&A *with* Mo

Q I am fairly active—I get to the gym 2 to 3 times a week—but I still have flabby upper arms. How do I tone them up?

A A lot of women in my classes complain about the flabby parts that hang from the bottom of their upper arms. I explain that this is in part due to excess body fat and lack of tone in muscle and skin tissue—and that can happen at any age and it's not always connected to being overweight. To get rid of it, you have to do both cardiovascular and strength-training exercises. Cardiovascular exercise (such as Newbody or any aerobic-based activity that vigorously incorporates swinging "running" arms—for example, power walking, walking uphill, or fast jogging) helps burn fat all over the body and tone the upper-arm muscles and shoulders. As for strength training, you'll need to do targeted training especially for the triceps, like push-ups. The Newbody workout and Newbody Extra Strength A routine will give you everything you need to develop shape and strength in every muscle of your upper body—in just 15 minutes! No more saggy arms for you!

5

Newbody Chest

Years ago, my girlfriend Pat and I decided to start running together twice a week in the mornings before work. She lived nearby and it seemed like an easy way to get outside more and spend some time together. In the middle of our third run, in between her huffing and puffing, Pat suddenly stopped and said, "You know, Mo, my heart's just not in it. I hate running."

The trouble is, her heart *was* in it. Any type of aerobic exercise—where you make yourself breathe hard and sweat—involves the heart and does all kinds of good things for it.

Pat and I decided to finish our "run" that day by walking—and talking about the types of physical activities that Pat might enjoy more. We quickly determined that running wasn't her sport. She told me she loved walking to and from her work every day and she liked group fitness—she had been on sports teams throughout her life.

So let's try fitness power walking instead, I suggested. And I also invited her to the Newbody class.

Today, Pat's heart is still in it 100 percent! We actually kept up our fitness walks and talks (and eventually runs) for almost a year (and having a fitness buddy that lived nearby was fabulous)—until I moved to the south end of the city. She loved the fact that Newbody was a combination of low-impact aerobic fitness and strength training, and today she still enjoys doing Newbody when her schedule allows her to come to my class on Wednesdays.

WEIGHT TRAINING FOR YOUR HEART AND CHEST

Your heart is a strong muscular pump that weighs between 7 and 15 ounces and is a little larger than the size of your fist. The heart sits between your lungs in the middle of your chest, behind and slightly to the left of your breastbone. It beats on average 100,000 times a day to pump blood throughout the body and deliver oxygen to every single cell. When experts recommend exercise for your heart, they're talking about consistent aerobic exercise (the kind that makes you breathe harder and increases your heart rate) for 20 to 30 minutes or longer. The overall objective of that exercise is to build the heart muscle so it pumps more efficiently (more blood is pumped per beat to create "greater stroke volume"). When you're in good shape, you have a lower resting heart rate. While 77 beats per minute is around normal for the average adult population, elite athletes can have heart rates in the 40s or low 50s. I'm not asking you to be an elite athlete by any means. But following my Newbody program *will* strengthen your heart and lower your resting heart rate some. And that preserves heartbeats for a long and healthy life.

Your chest includes some of the largest muscle groups in the upper body. The chest muscles—pectorals (major and minor)—are responsible for lifting the upper limbs and bringing them across the body. These muscles are large muscles that help give shape and tone to your chest. Large muscles can handle more weight, which allows you to burn more calories. While you burn up to 35 percent more calories when you simultaneously work the muscles in your upper and lower body during a workout, lean muscle also continues to burn a lot of calories even at rest! As wonderful as aerobic exercise is for your heart, strength training has just as many benefits. Some of the most common chest exercises include push-ups, chest presses, and chest flies. The benefits? You're going to have a toned and shapelier chest and maybe perkier breasts! You will have a stronger chest so you can push a lawnmower, move the fridge (or any heavy piece of furniture), push and pull the door of your car open and closed, push yourself out of bed every morning, and pick yourself up off the floor if you should fall! All this new-found strength also comes with a huge boost of confidence and a feeling of satisfaction and happiness with yourself and the world! Now who's going to argue with that?

THE HEART-RATE TRAINING ZONE

To get the most out of aerobic exercise and keep it safe, monitor your intensity throughout your workouts to ensure that you're working within your heart-rate training zone and getting a good workout. You don't want to burn out by working too hard, and you don't want to get frustrated because you're not working hard enough—and not seeing results.

Finding your target heart-rate zone

The target heart-rate zone is the pulse rate (in beats per minute) that allows you to exercise safely while getting the maximum benefits from your workout. This range is usually between 60 and 80 percent of your maximum heart rate.

First, find your maximum heart rate by subtracting your age from 220. To calculate 60 to 80 percent of your maximum heart rate, multiply that number by 0.6, or 60 percent, to get your lower exercise range and by 0.8, or 80 percent, to get your higher exercise range.

When you take your pulse while exercising, it should be between the lower and upper numbers. If it's below, you need to work harder; if it's higher, determine how you're feeling and lower the intensity if need be.

Of course, if you have a medical condition (for example, high blood pressure), your heart rate should stay below a certain level. It is always important to speak with your physician before beginning any exercise program.

Monitoring your heart rate

You can monitor your heart rate in a few different ways:

- At the gym, most cardiovascular machines measure your heart rate for you with built-in sensors.
- Purchase a heart-rate monitor.
- Manually, take your pulse at the wrist or neck using the first two fingers (index and middle). Every 5 or 10 minutes, find your pulse, look at the clock, and count beats for 15 seconds. Multiply this number by 4 to determine your heart rate.

Using the rate of perceived effort scale

Another way to calculate how hard you're working is to use the simple scale below. It measures your rate of perceived effort. Typically, you want to be scoring a 5 to 7 on the scale during your workout (you can talk in sentences, your heart- and breathing rates are elevated, and you're breaking a sweat but able to maintain) and aim for between 7 and 8 (you're feeling the effort, your breathing is heavier, you can feel your heart pounding, and you're sweating and pushing the aerobic-anaerobic threshold). When you reach 8 and higher, typically you're breathless and can't talk and breathe at the same time—this is anaerobic training and you won't be able to maintain this level of intensity longer than 15 to 45 seconds, depending on your fitness level.

0	Nothing at all
1	Very, very light
2	
3	Fairly light
4	
5	Moderate
6	
7	Somewhat hard
8	Hard
9	
10	Very hard

NEWBODY TIP: It's not only what you do that's going to save your heart and your life, it's what you eat and how you prepare your food—making heart-healthy choices in the kitchen. With this in mind, I have created my Newbody Sensible Eating Plan (see page 189) to help you lose or manage your ideal weight and get the body you desire—and to give you all the nutritional tools to take care of your heart! Making heart-healthy choices is easier than you might think. Lose the salt shaker, load up on vegetables and fruits, and choose healthy fats and whole grains. Follow my 5 P's Please program (see page 192) and your heart will love it.

EXERCISE YOUR HEART

Like the other muscles in your body, your heart needs to stay active to stay fit and healthy. Health Canada recommends at least 30 minutes of physical activity at a moderate to somewhat hard intensity level most days to achieve and maintain good health. Anyone with a heart condition should talk to their doctor before starting an exercise program. Here's how aerobic exercise can benefit your heart:

- **IT STRENGTHENS YOUR HEART AND CARDIOVASCULAR SYSTEM**—and that means your heart is working as efficiently as possible, whether you're working out, walking with your kids to the store, or running downstairs to watch a TV show that started 5 minutes ago!

- **IT LOWERS CHOLESTEROL.** Regular exercise helps raise the level of good cholesterol (HDL cholesterol) in your blood. HDL helps remove the bad cholesterol (LDL cholesterol) from your arteries. (On the other hand, a high level of LDL in the blood can cause fatty build-up in your arteries—which blocks the flow of blood and is a risk factor for causing a heart attack).

- **IT HELPS LOWER YOUR RESTING HEART RATE.**

- **IT REDUCES YOUR BLOOD PRESSURE.** Exercise makes your heart stronger, and a stronger heart can pump more blood with less effort—which lowers blood pressure. Blood pressure is the pressure exerted by circulating blood on the walls of blood vessels. Over time, high blood pressure strains the heart and eventually weakens it.

- **IT LOWERS YOUR WEIGHT.** Regular exercise plays a key role in achieving healthy weight goals—whether you're maintaining a healthy weight or losing weight. Being overweight makes your heart work really hard all the time, which increases the risk of heart disease and can raise blood pressure and cholesterol levels. Regular exercise burns calories and helps you lose weight. Losing weight takes the load off the heart.

- **IT EASES YOUR BREATHING.** Keep in mind that, as you train your heart, your lungs are getting trained too! The heart and lungs work in harmony to provide oxygen and other nutrients to the cells throughout your body.

- **IT COMPENSATES FOR REDUCED HORMONE LEVELS.** It's a well-known fact that estrogen protects women from developing certain types of heart disease. Before menopause, it decreases our risk of having a heart attack—men have a much higher risk of heart attack because they don't have estrogen. After menopause, a woman's estrogen level falls, and by age 60, men and women have approximately the same risk. But here's good news: regular exercise can step up to the plate to improve cardiovascular health as well as energy and weight management.

- **IT KEEPS YOU HAPPY.** Exercise can help reduce stress and depression, both of which are known to stress the heart. Work out your stress, and your heart will be happy and thank you!

Heart disease and women

Canadian women have caught up to men when it comes to the number of deaths from cardiovascular disease. One in every three Canadian women will die from heart disease or stroke—it is the number-one killer of all diseases for women. The Heart and Stroke Foundation says that females are more likely to die after a heart attack or stroke than males—and less likely to see a cardiologist after a heart attack. That's all the more reason to make regular activity a part of your life.

Sweat equity in your heart

Did you know that when you're worried about something adrenaline and other hormones get released into the blood? This is a physiological response designed to rouse the body for emergency action. Your heart pounds faster, muscles tighten, blood pressure rises, breath quickens, and your senses become sharper in order to prepare you to respond to what the body perceives as a physical danger. (That's how powerful our thoughts are!) This is called the "fight or flight" stress response, and in a lot of cases, it's useful because it really does help to motivate you or give you the energy to get things done. But when worry is chronic and you don't do anything about it (you just sit and stew), it can have detrimental effects on your health and specifically your heart, including depression, high blood pressure, and chest pains (angina). This is where exercise can make a difference. Moving your body is a great way to combat stress and worry. Regular exercise increases your tolerance to stress and allows you to manage your stress response better when you need to take some kind of action—and that's whether it's getting your house cleaned for surprise guests, running after your toddler as he or she heads the wrong way in the park, or hitting tight deadlines at work so that you can get to your Newbody class on time.

Breathe ... it's heartfelt

Studies have shown that activities that focus on slowing down and regulating the breath may help to decrease the risk of heart disease—because slow, deep breathing helps you relax, and when you're relaxed and calm, your heart rate slows down. Meditation involves sitting quietly and focusing on something such as your breath, an object, or a mantra, to calm your thoughts and relax. A lot of yoga classes use various forms of meditation and deep breathing. While a formal class is terrific, I've developed a quick and simple breathing exercise that I can use anywhere and anytime to calm myself down. For example, if I'm rushing to an important meeting I will often sit in my car for a few minutes before heading in and do this exercise. Simply sit quietly for 1 minute and focus on taking slow, long, deep breaths. This is a great way to calm down. Here's a longer relaxation exercise that is called a *body scan*. Try it at home. Some people like to do a body scan when they go to bed.

- Lie on your back with your legs out, arms by your sides with the palms up. Your eyes can be open or closed. Take several deep breaths.
- As you begin to feel relaxed, direct your attention to the toes of your left foot. Tune in to any sensations for 10 to 30 seconds while remaining aware of your breathing. Now focus your attention to the toes of your right foot.
- Move your focus to the sole of your left foot and hold it there while continuing to pay attention to your breathing. Switch to the sole of your right foot.
- Follow the same procedure as you move to your ankles, calves, knees, thighs, hips, and so on, moving up the body. Spend at least 5 minutes, longer if you can. Pay particular attention to any areas where you may be feeling discomfort or even pain. Also pay particular attention to the head: the jaw, chin, lips, tongue, roof of the mouth, nostrils, throat, cheeks, eyelids, eyes, eyebrows, forehead, temples, and scalp.
- When you're finished, go back to focusing on only your breath. Focus on breathing in and out for a few minutes. Then slowly open your eyes and move your fingers and toes. You should feel fabulous!

REDUCE THE RISK OF BREAST CANCER

Breast cancer statistics are scary: one in nine women in Canada will develop breast cancer in her lifetime. But studies show that even moderate physical activity may reduce your risk for breast cancer by 30 to 40 percent! Health Canada recommends aerobic exercise or activities (that should make you sweat and breathe harder) for at least 30 minutes on 5 or more days of the week. Aerobic exercise (good examples are brisk walking and Newbody workouts) will also help you lose excess weight. Being overweight by more than 11 pounds is associated with increased breast cancer risk too, especially among postmenopausal women. I recommend that every woman exercise not only for her heart but for her breasts!

Q&A *with* Mo

Q I've heard that when women lose weight, they often lose it from their breasts first. I'm not that well endowed to begin with—is there any way I can avoid this?

A Great question. Unfortunately, since breasts are mostly fatty tissue, they are the first to go when the body becomes lean. But here's the good news: including weight training in your regular exercise program will help firm up the muscles that support the breast tissue, giving the appearance of perkier breasts. In fact, I tell my class that exercises that focus on the pectoral muscles beneath the breasts are almost as good as a fancy underwire bra because stronger muscles there will lift breasts. There are other things you can do to lessen the appearance of sagging:

1. Be aware of your posture—in and out of the gym. Posture goes a long way toward elongating your appearance and contributing to a higher look for your breasts.
2. Wear a supportive bra, especially a sport bra when exercising. Make sure your bras are comfortable and the correct size. While wearing a bra doesn't do anything to firm your muscles, it does create a pleasing outline, and when you wear one that flatters your figure, your breasts are lifted in an attractive way.

6

Newbody Back

Eighty percent of the population will have a back problem sometime in their life. And I know, as a registered physiotherapist and fitness professional, that 60 percent of that back pain could be solved simply by moving your body more and by doing aerobic exercise and functional forms of strength training on a regular basis—which is what the Newbody program is all about!

Moving your body regularly helps you consistently burn more calories daily (which helps you lose weight), stop slouching, and stand tall and proud. Sedentary pursuits, on the other hand, such as watching endless hours of TV and being stuck working at a desk or staring at a computer screen all day long tend to bring about unhealthy postural habits—for example, poking your head and chin forward, rounding your shoulders and upper back, flattening your lumbar curve, and sticking your belly out. That not only sounds dreadful, it feels painful.

For women, low- and mid-back pain are the most common complaints, but chronic neck pain is also prevalent with increasing levels of stress in our lives. Low-back pain is most often brought on by poor posture and sedentary living (lack of adequate exercise). Layered on top of that is the complaint of mid-back pain, which sometimes occurs in women due to pressure from their bra straps (both on the shoulders and where your bra straps rests on your spine). Surprised? Don't be: it's very common. We learn to ignore the pressure and eventually those pressure points become numb.

What happens is that you adapt your posture in response to the pressure, and eventually your back becomes stiff and/or painful.

Being overweight or obese puts even more load on the spine and can exacerbate back problems. This is another good reason to lose weight—and there's no better way than by getting active and making healthier and more sensible food choices. By combining the two, you will be easily able to lose 500 calories (250 calories with my Newbody program and 250 with my Newbody Sensible Eating Plan) and lose at least 1 pound of fat weight a week. That's a healthy weight loss!

Keep in mind that if you're sedentary, it's not how much you do, it's how you do it. In order to be safe and effective, exercise must be mindful and smart. Investing in professional help—such as joining a fitness club, hiring a personal trainer, and investing time to follow the advice in this book—is a good idea because you'll learn what to do and how to exercise safely.

POWER UP YOUR POSTURE: LIFT AND TUCK, SQUEEZE AND BREATHE

- Lift your heart to open (expand) your chest. This will automatically lengthen your spine and lift your head. Your goal is to position your head directly over your neck and shoulders. Naturally, most of us allow our chins to poke forward, which is the cause of poor posture, especially when we sit all day at work. But if you lift your chest, then subtly tuck your chin in, you will position your head over your neck and be looking ahead without feeling tension in your neck. Also, by lifting your chest first, your shoulders will move back, making it easier to squeeze the muscles that set the shoulders in proper position.
- Squeeze the muscles between and beneath the shoulder blades to draw the shoulders down (away from your earlobes) and slightly in, toward the spine. If you stand or sit all day, or experience a lot of stress in your life, you most likely will find your shoulders lifted and rounded forward. You may also notice that as you've become older, your posture has become rounded and even your breasts appear to sag. Change your head and shoulder posture while you watch yourself in the mirror. You

will see youthfulness and energy return as you lift your chest (step 1), and squeeze your mid-back and shoulder girdle muscles (step 2).

- Tuck your abdominals in by gently pulling your belly button toward your spine. It is more of an inward and upward tuck rather than a "suck," as we used to say and do. Think of performing this exercise the same way as you would perform the Heimlich manoeuvre with your fists—but instead, get your navel to move in and up. This will activate your deeper abdominals like a muscle "corset." This will also lift your pelvis upward (hips toward ribs) just enough to level your hips (pelvis) into neutral (that is, not tilted forward or back). You only want to tuck your belly button in and up with 50 percent of your total effort. You should be able to breathe and there should be a natural curve (inward) in your lower back. This is the most common muscle imbalance that leads to back pain, and in part it is due to poor posture associated with weak abdominals. In addition, excess body weight sits around the belly and makes matters worse. Changing the way you stand and sit is a great start.
- Squeeze your gluteal muscles (buttocks) to stabilize your pelvis. As with your abdominals, only squeeze your gluteals about 50 percent of your total effort so that they are gently contracting. Imagine holding a lottery ticket between your buttocks when you're standing, walking, and even exercising. This is a motivating visual image. Squeezing your gluteals serves another very important function for women. It helps you align your thigh bone (femur) correctly so that as you squat, lunge, step, walk, leap, jump, and run, you have a better chance of keeping your knee in better alignment, and thus minimizing the impact stresses on that joint (as well as the lower back). This squeeze is key to improving your exercise technique. I often coach class participants to "squeeze your gluteals (buttocks)" in every exercise for the lower body. Not only will you improve your posture, but you will get a better butt as a result!
- My final points on posture: to help align your spine and achieve powerful posture, keep your knees slightly bent and feet positioned on the ground just wider than hip width. If you're squeezing your gluteals as instructed, then your feet should be

slightly turned out. When you walk, your toes should point almost directly forward. When you stand powered up in your posture, you will almost instantly feel lighter, look slimmer by 5 to 7 pounds, and even appear more confident. You will likely find yourself making better eye contact with people simply because you are standing tall with your head high.

NEWBODY TIP: Place sticky notes around your house with a smiley face symbol (☺) to remind yourself to stand and sit in good posture. I have one on my computer screen, steering wheel, and front hall mirror. This has got to be one of the most effective behaviour modification tools I have ever created for myself. When you see the smile, it reminds you what you need to do—and it makes you smile back. When I shared this with my back patients in the 1980s they loved it and so did I. I didn't have to nag at them to correct their posture. I just gave them a grin or a sticky note with a ☺!

INSTANT BACK RELIEF

- Stop several times during your day to take a few deep breaths to expand the ribs, release muscle tension, and align your spine. Learn how to power up posture. When you're sitting at your desk or in a meeting or driving your car, check to see that you're sitting up tall and that your shoulders are relaxed and down away from your ears. If you can take deep, expansive breaths without too much effort, you're likely in good alignment.
- Wear a properly fitted bra so pressure from the bra straps is minimal. A front-closing bra or bra without a closing clasp may help.
- Do sloppy push-ups that don't require you to be strong. Here's how: start in a regular push-up position, lying on your stomach with your forearms on the ground alongside your ribs and hands placed (with palms down) just wider than your shoulders. Push your chest up from the floor slowly as you breathe in. Keep your eyes gazing down, chin tucked in, and hips down on the floor. It's not how high you go that makes this stretch so effective—it's how relaxed you keep your trunk and lower body. The work is in your arms. Push up onto your forearms to start, pause to exhale, and as you breathe in, lower yourself down to

the floor. Repeat 5 to 10 times at a slow, comfortable pace. (It will take some time, but as you get stronger in your arms and more flexible in your spine, you may be able to push up until your arms are almost extended—but still keep your elbows bent and hips on the ground.)

- Give yourself a hug each day to open and stretch your upper and lower back. You can do this simply by wrapping your arms around in front and reaching for the opposite shoulder. Hold and breathe in, then gently pull your shoulders as you exhale. If you wish to stretch the lower back in the same way, lift and hug one knee at a time, then switch sides. When you lie down to go to sleep, hug both knees to your chest and gently draw your chin in to lengthen the neck and the spine. Hold for a few deep, slow breaths; release and repeat. Give your back some love with a hug throughout the day.

BUILD A BETTER BACK

Women always want to strengthen and tone targeted areas: their chest, abdominals, thighs, triceps, and butt, which are the areas that tend to soften and sag with age. But "oh my aching back, I don't dare." Most women don't think a lot about the muscles they don't see as often in the mirror or the muscles they don't really know how to strengthen and stretch—and for the majority of the population, those are the muscles in the back. Your back muscles are so important and they *need* your attention. If you really want a new body, you'll need to embrace back training, and that is why I have scheduled the Extra Strength C (core) routine 3 times per week. This will ensure that you build a stronger, better back and protect yourself against injury. To get a new body, you must have a strong back!

To build a better back, it's important to train the back muscles in the way we need those muscles to work every day. We need our back muscles to support us when we are sitting at our desk, walking to the store, bending and lifting, twisting and reaching, and exercising. In the back-friendly Newbody program, we do the entire 30-minute program on our feet. While we are exercising, we use our back muscles functionally to keep us in proper position and balanced.

Doing low-impact aerobic activities is a great way to begin strengthening your back (and abdominal muscles) and improve your posture and body awareness naturally. Low-impact aerobic exercise and specific strengthening exercises tone the muscles that support the back without causing undue strain on the important structures that are most vulnerable to stress. These include the sacrum and lumbar vertebrae and intervertebral discs. Besides strengthening muscles, low-impact aerobic exercise increases bone density. Walking, elliptical striding, cycling, swimming, and cross-country skiing are great examples of low-impact exercise that provide great cross-training activity. You can add them into your fitness plan as you like.

Aerobic exercise in general will also help with weight-loss goals, if that's important, and losing weight will help relieve back pain, especially lower back pain. Aerobic activities also help increase circulation and relieve muscle tension and back pain by relieving stress. The good news is that you don't have to go hard in intensity to benefit. Moderate intensity (5 to 6 RPE) is all that you need to lower your stress, and as you build your fitness over time, you can also build your energy and stamina.

Bone up on weight-bearing forms of exercise. A new body begins with a strong and stable foundation—your bones. With the right balance in strength training (2 to 3 times a week) and good nutrition, your skeleton will support your back for years to come. At menopause, estrogen levels drop dramatically, causing women to lose bone density faster than ever—at a rate of 2 to 5 percent each year. Active and athletic women have 5 to 30 percent better bone mineral density than non-active women.

Do dynamic exercises in moderation to ensure that you're delivering enough force through your bones to stimulate bone mineralization and maintain bone density. These types of activities include running and running-based activities, jumping rope (skipping), as well as mixed-impact, step-training, or martial arts–based fitness classes. You can do even higher intensity (low-repetition) resistance training once you reach your Newbody goal. Higher impact activity is good for you and necessary for strong bones, as long as your body is fit to withstand the impact stresses.

Say "good morning" to your back

To reduce your risk of lower-back or disc injury or degeneration, you should not repeatedly flex (bend forward from the waist) your lumbar spine in the first 60 to 90 minutes after waking up. The intervertebral discs are fully hydrated from lying down all night. That's not a bad thing (it's also one of the reasons you are tallest in the morning—the discs deflate during the day), but it means that when you bend over to tie up your shoes first thing, you'll likely feel pretty stiff unless you bend your knees. Warm up your body and your back before engaging in more intense aerobic activity or more specific trunk exercises, as this is the easiest way to protect your back and discs.

If you like to work out first thing in the morning, the Newbody program is perfectly safe because you are on your feet and there is little to no trunk flexion involved. There are very few exercises in the Extra Strength routines that flex the trunk (the exception is the abdominal crunches and cycles, so I would encourage you to leave those until the end of the workout when your body and back will be ready to handle the effort). Also remember that no matter what time of day it is, if any exercise bothers your back, then "back off." Check your technique, decrease your range of movement, or avoid it altogether. Finish your day with flexibility stretches to release the tension in your muscles from your day or to complement the stretching that you did in your workout. Your back will appreciate any and all stretching that you do for it.

Give your back a break

- Work out back kinks: sit on a chair with knees bent and feet flat on the floor, and bend forward at the hips. Bend your arms behind you, with palms facing away from you, and make fists. Knead circles into your lower back on either side of your spine. Continue working your way up for a minute or more. Find a good massage therapist and treat yourself to a 30-minute basic neck or back massage. You don't even have to lie down or take off your clothes.

- Strengthen your back by strengthening your abdominals. The muscles that criss-cross your midsection weave through your torso and attach to your spine. When your abdominal muscles are weak, the muscles in your butt and legs compensate for the work your abs should be doing. This destabilizes the spine and eventually leads to back pain and strain. Develop a strong core to avoid these problems. (See the Newbody Extra Strength C routine for all the best core exercises to build a better back.)

- Exercises that work the muscles of your mid-back—as well as the muscles of your rear shoulders—will improve your posture, prevent you from hunching, and give the illusion of a firmer bustline. Dead lifts and bent-over rows are winners!

- Wear supportive, comfortable footwear. I'm not saying never wear sexy high heels, but love and respect your feet most of the time. They are your body's connection to the earth. Comfortable and supportive footwear with proper arch support and cushioning will help support your tootsies. This will set the foundation for correct alignment of the spine.

- Sleep healthfully. Your time asleep is when the body rests and repairs itself. A minimum of 6 to 8 hours a day is best. How you sleep is also quite important. If you sleep on your side, a pillow between your legs helps support your back. Proper pillow size should also be considered, to help keep the head in alignment with the rest of the spine.

- Always maintain good posture. Incorporate my sticky-note reminders to help you sit and stand properly. Practice makes posture perfect. Sitting up straight is a sure way to keep your spine aligned and stress on your back at a minimum. If you have not paid attention to your posture for some time, start paying attention by incorporating some or all of my healthy back tips into your day and your self-care. They each take 1 minute or less to do. Adopt my sticky-note message reminders to sit and stand up straight. Consciously practise—start with 30 seconds a day (or while you brush your teeth) and build up to 5 minutes at a time. Eventually you should be able to sit up straight for 1 minute every hour of the day. Get up and walk to the water fountain or look out your office window while you're on the phone. This makes it easy to straighten up; before long you will find that sitting up straight will be no more complicated than taking a walk or reading a book.

- Exercise regularly. Newbody gets you exercising 6 times a week! Always keep in mind that exercise is great medicine for your back, body, and mind. It helps relieve stress, support sleep, keep bones strong, improve muscle strength ... the benefits go on and on.

- Keep your core muscles strong and working together to support your back. You need to train your abdominals, back, hips, and shoulder girdle muscles together to ensure that they can work together in your daily life. You will know how effective you are—if you remain back pain- and injury-free, you're doing something right. My Newbody program and Extra Strength routines will get you there and keep you going!

Three Ms for bone health

This is an easy way to remember how to keep your bones healthy:

1. **MAXIMIZE BONE DENSITY.** Building strong bones during childhood and adolescence can be the best defence against developing osteoporosis later. A healthy lifestyle, including regular exercise and a balanced diet, gives children a great start.

2. **MAINTAIN BONE DENSITY.** By their mid-30s, women begin to lose bone density. Be sure you get enough calcium and vitamin D to slow down bone loss *and* keep investing in a healthy lifestyle.

3. **MINIMIZE BONE LOSS.** We naturally lose bone density as we grow older. But at menopause, estrogen levels drop dramatically, causing women to lose bone density faster than ever—at a rate of 2 to 5 percent each year. A healthy lifestyle helps to minimize this loss.

Q&A *with* Mo

Q Why do some women shrink in size as they get older? And is that going to happen to me?

A Shrinking in height is usually caused by a loss of bone cells in the spine (osteopenia) as well as a loss of lean muscle mass, strength, and flexibility. While these are natural changes, there are lifestyle habits that can help you prevent it from happening. Women need to bone up on exercise and eat a healthy diet that includes rich forms of high-quality calcium, and the sooner in life you do that (within the first 16 years of your life when bones are forming is most important), the more you will preserve your bones for life. Just about every cell in the body relies on calcium to function properly. Calcium is a fat-burning nutrient too, so once you enter menopause and your estrogen declines, the need for calcium rises to help preserve bone cells from loss. The body absorbs calcium directly from food, and it will steal calcium from bones if there's not enough available in the diet (when that happens, the bones become more porous, brittle, and more fragile).

To keep my bones strong (and not shrink to the size my mother did!) I exercise, eat healthily, and also take a good multivitamin and mineral supplement that includes high-quality calcium, phosphorous, magnesium, zinc, folic acid, vitamins A, K, B6, and B12. I get outside for at least 30 minutes a week (my running time) for a healthy dose of vitamin D (from sunlight), which is harder to do in the winter months. I am also very mindful of foods that contain the calories, lean protein, and essential nutrients necessary to ensure that I absorb enough calcium. There are a lot of calcium-rich foods to choose from, including low-fat dairy products, calcium-fortified soy, orange juice, and other beverages, some vegetables (especially dark green, leafy ones), fish products (those that contain bones, such as canned salmon and sardines), and meat alternatives (if you're like me and hate sardines). Lentils and beans contain calcium too.

One last note: calcium loss is increased by the consumption of excess salt, caffeine, alcohol, and protein—and that's why I say everything in moderation!

7

Newbody Abdominals

No matter where I am teaching or training in the world, women always ask me what is the best exercise they can do to flatten their tummies—and they're always surprised when I tell them it's not crunches. Far from it. Today, crunches are only one small part of an efficient strengthening program for abdominal muscles. In fact, the best way to flatten that tummy is to do functional exercises such as the plank exercise on page 172 (see Newbody Tip) and the plank variations in the Extra Strength C routine, which target *all* the abdominal muscles around the core and mimic what the abdominals have to do every day.

The primary responsibility of the abdominal muscles is to move and stabilize your spine (in neutral) as you stand, bend, extend, twist, and move your body. It's important to train your abdominals in the way you use these muscles. In a typical day, you will sit and stand, bend over, lift, and twist to move your body long before you lie down on your back (to sleep at night). So it's best to train your abdominals in an upright position!

That's where Newbody's core training comes in. It helps you strengthen all the muscles that stabilize your body and hold your spine in a neutral position. (That's why I like to think of the abdominals as the glue that holds us still so we can move our arms, legs, and bodies.)

I keep saying "abdominals" because there is more than one muscle involved. While crunches primarily target one of four abdominal muscles (it's called the rectus abdominis) and work it in one direction, core training involves not only the other 3 abdominal muscles but also the back (spinal) muscles and some of the hip and shoulder muscles as well. To achieve a flat tummy, you must train your abdominals in their natural habitat along with their core friends. Together they will effectively support and align the spine, and make movements of the arms, upper body, legs, and lower body more efficient and powerful. Think of the golf swing. To have a long drive (and potentially low score, which is what you want), you need both stability and strength in the core to create a powerful swinging action.

Pilates exercise gets the credit for bringing the concept of core training into the spotlight. Pilates, named after its founder, Joseph Pilates, is a total conditioning program that works your body by focusing on core muscles and using your breath to help control the movements. It's a fabulous method of muscle strengthening that actually started as rehabilitation for dancers.

We use a lot of the same principles in Newbody, as we train the core to work and support the spine the way it needs to be supported in our daily life. You'll see that we stand tall as we move our feet and lift our legs (to march, skate, squat, and lunge forward, backward, and side to side) and move our torso and arms (bend and lift and twist, reach, pull, and press). You always have to be aware of keeping your abdominal muscles pulled in and held throughout the activity. I often say it's like wearing a corset—gradually pulling the strings of the corset tighter to support your back. The Newbody Extra Strength C routine is a 15-minute sequence devoted to the core too, so you can strengthen your abdominals and other core muscles (including your back) in a variety of positions and against gravity to help you get stronger faster.

Last but not least, the aerobic exercise aspect of my program also helps burn calories—and fat—to uncover your beautiful Newbody abs. Although you can't spot-reduce if you have an extra layer or two of fat over your abdominals, you can lose it by burning calories. I mix in the Extra Strength C routine often throughout each week because your core has to be as strong as possible to help you do the Newbody workout and the Extra Strength routines for 30 minutes, 6 days a week, without back pain and injury.

BELLY FAT: MEASURING YOUR HEALTH RISKS

Many health experts are now measuring people's waist circumferences as part of their annual checkup. That's because research shows that too much fat around the waist (that's the "apple" body shape) can lead to greater health risks for conditions including type 2 diabetes, heart disease, and even some types of cancer. Research by Health Canada and the World Health Organization indicates that women whose waists measure more than 35 inches and men whose waists measure more than 40 inches are at a greater risk of developing these health problems.

As you age, the amount of fat in your body often increases for a number of reasons—a slowing metabolism, stress, and hormonal imbalance. Women tend to put weight on in the belly area and you will see it. But there's more to belly fat than you can actually see and feel. The belly fat that lies deeper inside the abdomen and around your organs, including your heart (called visceral fat), has been linked to a higher risk of health problems such as heart disease and diabetes. Decreased physical activity, loss of lean muscle tissue, and heredity all contribute to overall weight gain for many people. Hormonal changes after menopause may also affect the way your body stores fat—leading to more fat in your belly.

You may not be able to change your genetic makeup, but you can change your metabolism, stress levels, hormonal responses, and activity level—and give your waistline a makeover.

Taking aim at belly fat is probably *the* most important health and anti-aging strategy that I recommend. Here are some tactics that will help reduce belly fat and manage your middle:

- **DRINK MODERATELY.** Avoid the "beer belly," and limit alcohol to no more than 1 drink a day (or 7 drinks a week).

- **STRETCH.** Sitting all day can tighten up and shorten the quadratus lumborum and psoas muscles, both of which act on the lower back to pull the spine out of proper alignment, which makes it tough to sit or stand up straight. Place one knee on a chair seat or bench (unweighted) and, keeping your hips straight, press your pelvis forward by squeezing your buttocks. Lift your chest and take a slow deep breath in and out. Lift your arm (the same side as your kneeling leg) up and over to toward the other side. Stay lifted through your spine. Do both stretches one after the other. Hold for 3 to 5 breaths each. Repeat on the other side.

- **BREATHE.** Feeling stressed can boost belly fat by increasing levels of cortisol, a hormone that sends fat to the tummy. Find a stress-buster that works for you and practise it daily. I like to stand in a hot shower, breathe in lavender and eucalyptus essential oils, and stretch, get out for a quick 15-minute walk or jog, and meditate in traffic jams (with my eyes open, of course).

- **SNACK HEALTHILY.** When you're feeling stressed, you're often inclined to snack on sweets for quick comfort—which sends more fat to the belly. Be prepared for those times by keeping healthy snacks on hand or going to the gym instead. A handful of almonds, an apple, or half a pita pocket with almond or peanut butter and sliced banana are three of my favourite stress-busting snacks.

- **TRY BELLYDANCING OR LATIN DANCING.** They focus on strengthening your core—and all that shimmying hip action is helpful and fun!

- **TAKE A YOGA CLASS OR TAI CHI.** Or learn to meditate. These mind–body activities may help you lose your belly because they help to reduce stress levels and rebalance hormones (the happy ones against the bad ones, especially cortisol).

- **DO 30 MINUTES OF MODERATE INTENSITY AEROBIC EXERCISE REGULARLY** (to burn fat) and strength train (to strengthen and tone, build more muscle, and boost your metabolism and burn more calories even at rest).

NEWBODY TIP: Walk the Plank, a fabulous core and abdominal exercise. Here's how to do it:

- Start on all fours (hands under your shoulders with elbows slightly bent and knees directly under your hips).

- Lift your navel up and in toward your spine and hold (this will keep your spine in a long and neutral position). Gently squeeze both your shoulder blades in and your buttocks to stabilize from both ends.
- Extend your legs out one at a time until both legs are straight, with only your hands and toes supporting you in a plank position. If this is too challenging, then lower both knees to the floor, bringing your hips down. Keep your spine straight and strong.
- Slowly lower yourself down to the ground onto the right forearm (elbow close to your side) and then the left. Hold in the plank position here and breathe (2 breaths).
- Hold for 20 to 30 seconds, breathing steadily. As you build endurance, aim to hold this pose for 60 seconds. Your body should form a straight line from your shoulders to your heels (or knees, if you modified the exercise). Pull your abdominals in and imagine you are trying to lift your belly button up and in toward your spine.
- Rest down on the floor and begin again from the hands and knees, lowering onto your left forearm, then the right.

METABOLISM MAGIC!

Metabolism is the rate at which your body burns calories—and your body burns calories all the time. A faster metabolism will help you burn more calories and lose more weight, if that's what you need to do. Keep in mind that your metabolism decreases 5 percent a decade after the age of 40 (which is one of the reasons why some women tend to put on weight as they get older). Here's how to keep yours fired up!

- Eat 5 to 6 healthy meals and snacks a day so you're constantly firing up your furnace—and burning calories. Keep well hydrated—drink six to eight 8-ounce (250 mL) glasses of water every day. When you don't drink enough, your body starts to store calories rather than burn them.
- Do aerobic exercise for a temporary boost. While different activities burn different quantities of calories, what's most

important is that you raise your heart rate and sustain the activity for at least 30 minutes every day.

- Regular weight training boosts metabolism for the long run because you're building lean muscle, which requires energy. Muscle burns more calories than fat, so the more muscle you build, the higher your resting metabolic rate will be. Muscles burn calories constantly—even at rest or while you sleep.

NEWBODY TIP: Regular eaters manage their energy and waistlines better:

- Always eat a balanced breakfast. This will set your metabolism into motion, help balance blood sugar, and provide the energy you need for exercise.
- Eat smaller meals more often throughout the day to sustain your energy and maintain your metabolism and your waistline.
- Fill up on nature's foods: eat vegetables and fruits with every meal or snack.
- Drink one 8-ounce (250 mL) glass of water 30 to 60 minutes before you exercise, then sip on one 8-ounce (250 mL) glass during your workout.
- Don't exercise on an empty stomach. Maintain a proper balance of complex carbohydrates, healthy fats, and lean choices of protein at each meal, or snack healthily throughout the day to maintain your energy and reduce cravings.

AT THE CORE

Have you done your Kegels today? These exercises strengthen the pubococcygeus muscles—by contracting and relaxing the muscles that form part of the pelvic floor. The pelvic floor muscles support the bladder and reproductive organs. Working them can help to increase abdominal muscle strength and improve hip and lower back stability. At the same time, Kegel exercises are also used to treat urinary incontinence, especially after pregnancy. Hormone changes can relax the pelvic floor muscles after menopause too. You can do Kegels just about anywhere—while travelling, at work, or during random moments of your day. No one will be aware that you're doing the exercises.

- First, identify the pelvic floor muscles involved by purposely stopping the flow of urine in midstream and then allowing the urine to flow again.
- Remembering what it felt like to control these muscles, try to contract them when you aren't in the washroom. Try visualizing your pelvic floor muscles moving in and up like being in an elevator. If your stomach muscles tighten, your pelvic muscles are not being exercised correctly.
- Tighten your pelvic muscles for 3 seconds and then relax them for 3 seconds.
- Repeat the Kegel exercises 10 to 30 times each session, and do at least 3 sessions a day.
- Keep your abdominal strength up and this will automatically increase the strength of your pubococcygeus muscles.

Sex and the core

Strong abdominal, lower back, and pelvic floor muscles provide stamina and strength in the bedroom. Also, when you're fit and toned and in shape, you feel good about your body and you feel good about yourself—and that's going to improve your sex life.

Here's how to keep your abs turned on anytime:

- When sitting in your car or at your desk, sit up tall and pull in your abs as you would at the start of a crunch—but don't crunch. Instead, sit up tall, relaxing your shoulders and your buttocks. Hold your abs in for 60 seconds at a time at least once every hour. If you stop feeling your abdominals working, pull in and hold again. This is more challenging than you might think. Try to imagine your navel is kissing your spine.
- Practise this exercise while brushing your teeth or standing in a lineup at the grocery store and eventually incorporate it into your walking and your workouts. The more you do it, the more core awareness you will develop.

Q&A *with* Mo

Q I've heard stress can contribute to belly fat—how does that work?

A Too much stress too often, combined with poor coping habits, may cause imbalances in the body, including the overproduction of the stress hormone cortisol. This hormone leads to weight gain of the most dangerous kind—belly fat! Cortisol is also associated with overeating and cravings for high-calorie, fatty, and sugary foods. While stress will always be a part of daily living, providing motivation and excitement to all the things we do, regular aerobic exercise will help reduce symptoms of chronic stress and rebalance the hormones associated with belly fat accumulation. Mindful exercise, such as yoga and Tai Chi, is highly effective as a stress management strategy.

8

Newbody Hips and Butt, Legs and Feet

HIPS AND BUTT

Every culture has different attitudes about the best size and shape for the buttocks. But no matter what the proportion preference, here's what really matters: you need strong gluteal muscles to support good posture, hip, and leg mobility. And gluteal muscles are beautiful!

Women should also understand the mechanics of the female pelvis. It is generally wider than a man's because it is designed for child-bearing. But this design also sets us up for muscle imbalances that can throw off spinal, hip, and even knee alignment. That's why it's so important to strengthen the gluteal muscles—they keep us upright and able.

Since the gluteals are some of your body's most powerful muscles and called into action on every move that you make with your lower body, it's important that we train them right. Almost every exercise within the Newbody program targets the gluteals because we're moving our legs the entire time—and moving forward and backward, side to side, and up and down will prevent the natural downward slide that your rear-end muscles tend to make as they weaken and atrophy. A muscular rear end not only looks better, but it also supports energetic and functional movement and increases strength, stability, and balance.

Hip, hip, hooray for strength training

Even postmenopausal women in their 50s, 60s, and beyond can increase their strength by as much as 75 percent and increase their hip and spine bone density by 1 percent with strength training 2 times a week alone. Newbody will put an end to gluteal muscles that have become weak and saggy!

Stability training for your hips

Stability training teaches certain muscles to work isometrically (without motion) while stabilizing a part of the body in a desired position. Whether stability training is done standing on one leg, sitting unsupported, or while working out, it results in increased muscular strength, endurance, functional mobility, and flexibility. It also helps to enhance nervous system activity, as well as your balance, core function, and postural alignment. It helps to lower risk of injury too.

The hip bridge is a fantastic stability-training exercise that prepares you for the side revolving bridge exercise on page 116. It will help strengthen gluteal muscles, restore muscle tone, add strength to your pelvic floor, and even provide therapeutic strengthening and stretching for your lower back.

- To start, lie flat on your back with your knees bent, feet positioned hip width apart and close to your hips, and arms relaxed at your sides.
- Pull in abdominal muscles 50 percent of the way to tilt the pelvis back slightly. Squeeze your gluteals to lift the hips. Initiating the movement with your pelvis, lift your hips upward off the ground while maintaining a neutral spine. Lift only as high as it takes for your body to form a straight line from your knees to your shoulders.
- Hold the bridge with your gluteals squeezed tight for 2 to 5 breaths.
- Lower your hips and return to starting position.
- Repeat 5 to 10 times.

Shaping your butt

No matter what size or shape—flat, square, apple, or pear—there are lots of moves that can help shape up your bottom line. Four of the best moves are

1. **WALKING LUNGES.** Stand with feet hip width apart, back straight with chest lifted, holding a weight in each hand. Step forward with your right foot, keeping your head up and the spine in a neutral position. Bend both the front and back knees 90 degrees to lower the hips toward the floor until the front thigh is almost parallel with the floor. The heel of the front foot should be kept down on the floor, with the knee directly over the centre of the foot. Push down through the front heel as you push off the back foot to bring your left foot forward to meet the right. Repeat the exercise starting with the left foot for 1 repetition. Repeat 15 to 30 times.

2. **BALANCING SQUAT.** Balance on the right foot, left knee bent with foot lifted a few inches off the floor in front. Keeping your back straight, slowly sit back into your right hip, bending your right knee about 45 degrees. Pause, then press into your right heel to stand up. A total of 10 to 15 repetitions for each side is recommended. Complete all reps, then switch sides. You can make it harder by holding a dumbbell in each hand or make it easier by resting your left toes on the floor and, if needed, using a chair or stool for balance.

3. **THE ELLIPTICAL TRAINER, OR TREADMILL ON AN INCLINE.** Working out on this stationary equipment tones and sculpts all the muscles in your butt without the impact. The treadmill is also good, but put it on an incline to boost the recruitment of the gluteal muscles and calorie burn while minimizing stress on the knees. Walk or run as if you were climbing up a moderately steep hill.

4. **DIVE IN.** Swim with a strong flutter kick, which puts the focus on the lower body—and specifically your gluteals!

NEWBODY TIP: "Cover your butt" by putting your workout clothes on as soon as you get up in the morning or home from work. This will increase your chances that you will get to your workout or get to the gym sometime during the day or the evening. Also monitor how your clothes are fitting, especially your pants, because this is your best indicator of how you are doing. Sometimes all you need to keep going is to see your pants fit better. If you are tight on time, do the Extra Strength B routine for building a better butt. Add more steps to your day and watch your bottom line improve.

LEGS AND FEET

Let me tell you about the power of intentional stepping. While we do intentional stepping exercise in the Newbody workout, the term *intentional stepping* also refers to the ability to push your tush out of a chair or off the couch in one motion—and get your feet to the street each day with "vim and vigour," as they say. To have this kind of energy (and to just sustain the energy you had when you were younger), you need 30 minutes of intentional movement (physical aerobic exercise) as part of your regular activities of daily living. Research supports these findings—you'll have a reported 20 percent more energy just by doing some intentional movement.

And that's exactly what we do in the Newbody workout. We focus on the large muscles in the legs and perform the most time-efficient, weight-bearing exercises to build muscle strength and tone as well as bone density and joint stability. Combining upper- and lower-body exercises (Newbody includes lots of arm movements too) will increase muscle recruitment and energy expenditure and improve your body awareness and skill execution. In the long run, this will improve your ability to get off the couch with more energy and stamina!

All the while, you're developing shapely, sexy legs too. You use your legs throughout the entire workout, working the larger muscles as well as multiple muscle groups at one time. You never stop moving! Forward-stepping works the quadriceps and hamstrings. Lateral and skating moves help to shape inner and outer thigh muscles (not to mention the derrière)! The workout is low impact as well as intentional in that the muscles have to work in a variety of ways (shortening, lengthening, and holding without movement) and they require help from muscles in the hips and core above too!

The result: strong, shapely legs and strong and stable hips and back.

Q&A *with* Mo

Q I am noticing as I get older that my butt seems to be losing its shape—even drooping a bit. Is there anything I can do to stop that?

A There sure is ... two things.

1. Strength train! What's interesting is that women are always afraid that if they lift weights or strength train, they will get big, bulky muscles—especially in the lower body. But here's one spot on the body where a little bulk would be welcome! More muscle here gives a rounder, perkier, and lifted derrière as well as stronger legs and a longer, more powerful stride! More muscle burns more calories of course! Your muscle work will pay off in the end.
2. Feed your body a combination of healthy sources of carbohydrates and protein. Carbohydrates boost energy in order to get you through your workout. Losing weight is achieved by making better, smarter calorie choices—such as eating complex carbohydrates like oatmeal for breakfast, half a whole-grain pita for lunch, or sweet potatoes for dinner. But always include a lean protein along with your carbs—1/2 cup (125 mL) of low-fat plain yogurt or skim milk, 3 ounces (75 g) of tuna, salmon, or chicken breast. Remember: you don't need to cut the carbs to get the new body you want. You *do* need to add protein to build and preserve muscle tone and shape.

GET A LEG-UP ON SCIENCE

Health Canada and the World Health Organization both support research that shows that moving your body 10,000 steps a day adds up to better health by helping to fight obesity, heart disease, diabetes, osteoporosis, forms of arthritis, and even some types of cancer. And it makes you look and feel fabulous!

How far is 10,000 steps? The average person's stride length is approximately 2.5 feet. That means it takes just over 2000 steps to walk 1 mile—and so 10,000 steps is close to 5 miles.

In a half-hour Newbody workout, you'll take about 2500 steps—and that's a great start toward reaching the daily goal of 10,000 steps. According to health sources, the average Canadian takes about 2000 steps a day. A reasonable goal for most people is to increase the average number of daily steps each week by 500 a day until you reach 10,000 steps.

Wearing a pedometer is an easy way to track your steps each day. Start by wearing the pedometer every day for 1 week. Put it on your belt or waistband near the front of your hipbone when you get up in the morning and wear it until bedtime. Record your daily steps in a log or notebook. By the end of the week, you'll know your average daily steps. You might be surprised how many (or how few) steps you get every day. The good news is that when you track your steps, you're empowered and inspired to take more. People who wear pedometers are more aware of the benefits of walking and more likely to exercise enough for good health. Research shows that when people track their steps, they expend more energy—at least 2000 steps more a day. Studies also show that those exercisers who wear pedometers are more compliant to their walking program or workout.

Some pedometers can even estimate the distance you cover or the number of calories you burn—now that's getting fancy!

Walk this way

How many steps have you taken today? Here are guidelines for adults:

No. of Steps	How Active You Are
< 5000	sedentary
5000–7499	minimally active
7500–9999	somewhat active
10,000	active
> 12,500	highly active

EXERCISE DESIGNED FOR A WOMAN

Besides the obvious, there are important differences between the structure of men's and women's bodies that affect us during exercise. One of the biggest differences is the pelvis. A woman's pelvis is broader than a man's, which means that the femur bones angle more medially. As a result, women's knee joints are closer toward the midline and can result in a knock-kneed stance. It's actually no surprise that knee pain, or patellofemoral stress syndrome, is very common among female exercisers. This alignment makes them more vulnerable to impact stress. The kneecap is prone to not track properly as the knee bends and straightens with movement. Instead, it tracks laterally, causing increased pressure on the joint and resulting in aching and tenderness around and under the kneecap. Sitting for long periods of time, walking, squatting, and walking down stairs can also aggravate the knees. Here are some ways to protect your knees:

- **SHED EXCESS POUNDS.** Simply walking around puts pressure equal to three to five times your body weight onto your knees. Toting around extra pounds makes the burden even worse and may accelerate wear and tear and lead to degeneration of the joint and osteoarthritis.

- **BALANCE STRENGTH AND FLEXIBILITY.** Both stretch and strength exercises are important to build up muscles around the thigh, both at the hip and the knee. But you need to strike a balance. The most important muscles to strengthen are the buttocks, hamstrings (back of thigh), and the adductors (inner thigh). The most important muscles to stretch are the abductors (outer thigh) and the quadriceps (front of the thigh).

- **CHOOSE KNEE-FRIENDLY ACTIVITIES!** Low-impact fitness classes, walking, rowing, cross-country skiing, and cycling are low-impact activities. Long or repetitive bouts of walking or running on the same side of the road (roads slope down on the sides) or high-impact exercises, such as running or hiking downhill, are tough on knees. To protect knees, strengthen the muscles around the knee, especially the hamstrings and the buttocks. Newbody shows you how. Modify the intensity when your knees need a break.

- **CHECK YOUR STANCE AND TECHNIQUE.** It's really important that women widen their stance wider than hip width during squats, lunges, marches, and other stationary standing exercises to ensure correct alignment of the femur and more efficient recruitment of the muscles during the exercise. When performing squats, stand with heels in and feet slightly turned out (picture yourself standing at 5 minutes to 1 o'clock on a clockface). Always squeeze your buttocks tight as you execute leg exercises (both in weight-bearing and non-weight-bearing exercises) to help maintain proper alignment of the knee over the ankle. This minimizes stress on the knee joint itself and increases muscle strength and stability around the knee.

Walk more

Have fun doing the Newbody workout but also try to increase your daily steps by walking an extra 30 minutes a week to start. Build up to 2 to 3 hours a week. Every bit adds up—here's how:

- Take a walk with your spouse, child, or a friend.
- Walk the dog or a neighbour's dog.
- Always take the stairs instead of the elevator.
- If you take an escalator, walk it.
- Park at the back of the lot (at work or the shopping mall).

- Better yet, walk to the store!
- Hide the TV remote—get up to change the channel.
- Window shop outside or in a mall.
- Plan a walking meeting or take your lunch break on the road.
- Walk over to visit a neighbour.
- Get outside to walk around the garden or neighbourhood.

LOW-IMPACT EXERCISE YIELDS HIGH REWARDS

While low-impact exercise is often described as "friendly," "gentle," and "light," don't for a second think that it's low intensity too. In fact, the Newbody workout is a great example of what low-impact exercise is—friendly and yet challenging exercise that is beneficial for the heart and lower body muscles. Low-impact exercise (which is when one foot is always in contact with the ground) can deliver the same cardiovascular benefits as high-impact exercise, as long as the effort is in the movement itself. But compared to high-impact exercise, it's less stressful on the weight-bearing bones and joints of the body.

The key to making low-impact exercise highly effective is to involve your entire body in what you're doing and move intelligently. Here's how you'll add intensity in your Newbody workout:

- **USE YOUR LEGS AS THE DRIVERS.** You'll rely on the large muscles of the lower body to perform repetitive movements involving the legs.

- **INCORPORATE UPPER-BODY MOVEMENTS SIMULTANEOUSLY.** Swinging your arms as you walk, pushing and pulling your arms as you perform a squat, and performing alternating arm curls with light hand weights as you perform an alternating step-up contribute to overall intensity and calorie burning.

- **CHANGE THE PACE—GO FASTER, THEN SLOWER, THEN MIX IT UP!** This will make the workout more challenging as your muscles work at different paces.

- **PERFORM MOVES WITH A LARGE RANGE OF MOTION TO INCREASE THE MUSCLE INVOLVEMENT AND INTENSITY.** For example, when you march in place, you make the move harder by bringing your knees up higher and reaching your arms over your head instead of up to shoulder level or pushing them out in front instead of leaving them at your sides.

- **INCLUDE MULTIPLE MUSCLE AND JOINT MOVEMENTS WITHIN THE LOWER BODY.** Almost all cardio activities do involve the lower body, but you can increase intensity in your low-impact workout by including movements such as squats and lunges that require muscle from the core, hips, and legs. You can also add walking lunges or side steps with squats to your usual walking workout and feel the intensity change immediately.

- **HOLD LIGHT WEIGHTS** and move with them to help recruit more muscle in the upper body and core—this can increase intensity by up to 30 percent.

HARDER—NOT HIGHER—IMPACT FOR WEIGHT LOSS

People who engage in higher intensity exercise over the long haul are the most successful at losing weight and keeping it off. The goal is to get your heart rate to the middle to high end of your heart-rate training zone—that is, 70 to 85 percent of your maximum training heart rate—and keep it there for at least 30 minutes, 3 or more times a week. This can be a tough order for someone who is just starting out in exercise, but the good news is that you don't have to do high-impact activities such as running hard and combat-style aerobic fitness classes in order to achieve this goal. Alternating your intensity level from moderate to high levels works very effectively. To elevate the heart rate and expend more calories, you have to move at a safe but quick pace while performing large leg movements repeatedly and involving as many other muscles as possible. The higher the intensity, the harder your heart and muscles will work and the higher number of calories you'll burn. As a result, you will be able to withstand working at a higher heart rate and your muscles will become stronger, more toned, and more metabolically active, which will drive up your energy needs (and the numbers of calories you burn) long after the workout is over! Doing this type of interval exercise—varying the intensity of exercise by going hard for 30 seconds to 1 minute, then going easy for 30 seconds to 1 minute, for 20 to 30 minutes at a time—will help you adapt more easily to higher intensity exercise.

High-impact exercise is safe as long as you are in the proper shape to tolerate the stresses on your bones and joints. Avoid higher impact activities if you

- Are new to exercise
- Are pregnant
- Have a joint injury or back pain
- Are significantly overweight
- Do not enjoy those forms of exercise

ACTIVATE YOUR FOOT MUSCLES

Try to do one of these exercises every day to activate foot muscles.

- **EASY FOOT MASSAGE.** Take a tennis ball, rolling pin, or foam roller and roll it under your foot. Do it slowly and make sure to include every part of the foot. Pay special attention to areas that are tender or sore as you perform the action. This is a great exercise to practise when you wake up or after a long day of work. You will also notice after performing this massage that you may even have more hamstring (back of your thigh) flexibility. Bend over and try to touch your toes. Do the massage and then try to touch again. You'll be able to go farther.

- **TOWEL EXERCISE.** Sit in a chair on a slippery surface, such as a linoleum floor. Place one foot on a small hand towel (with your toes in the middle and heel toward the back of the towel). While keeping your heel down, lift your entire foot, stretch your toes out, and lower them on the towel. Grab the towel with your toes and pull up through your arch to scrunch the towel up. Make sure your heel stays stable. Continue for 5 to 10 repetitions and then reverse. Curl the toes up and then straighten them out to spread the towel out on the floor. Repeat 5 to 10 times. Change feet and repeat. This is also a fabulous exercise to do while standing in the shower.

NEWBODY TIP: For happy and healthier feet, go "feet naked." Your feet need to be strong and flexible just as any other part of your body, and certain barefoot exercises are great way to exercise your feet. Have you ever taken a yoga or Pilates class? If you have, then you know how effective these types of workouts can be for your feet and your body. Strengthening the 33 muscles of your foot will help improve your balance, strength, and posture.

Q&A *with* Mo

Q I've noticed that the skin on my legs is not as firm as it used to be. I am 52, in good shape, and still exercise 3 to 5 times a week! What gives?

A Unfortunately as we age we lose proteins in our skin (called collagen and elastin) and estrogen in our bodies. When that happens, the elasticity, bounciness, and resiliency of skin suffers. Active and leaner women notice this change all over their bodies, but it is especially noticeable on their legs. Keep doing your aerobic conditioning and strength-training exercises though—to stay at a healthy weight and to help tone the skin and the muscle underneath and reduce the appearance of "saddle bags" and even cellulite. Be sure to drink eight to ten 8-ounce (250 mL) glasses of water and eat a nutritiously rich and balanced diet each day. Hydrating moisturizers—natural plant extracts with essential oils—can make a visible difference, and massage therapy increases circulation to the skin, loosens up tight muscles, and relaxes your whole body. You might also choose workout leggings that cover up a bit more leg, such as capris. Your legs and your feet support you all day long—be sure to treat them with tender loving care.

9

The Newbody Sensible Eating Plan

There is no secret, diet, or magic pill that will help you lose weight. When it comes to achieving healthy weight loss, it's all about getting back on track with the basics—sensible eating and exercise. I'm not saying it's easy, especially in the beginning, but when you make a conscious choice to do something and then do it consistently, you'll be able to transform your body and your health. You'll be able to lose the excess, stubborn pounds and begin to build your new body. By choosing to feed your body with nutrient-rich foods throughout the day to sustain energy and balance blood sugar levels, you'll be able to exercise and build your fitness level, shape up your metabolism, satisfy food and hunger cravings, and rebalance your hormones. By following my Newbody Sensible Eating Plan, you'll cut calories, eat less fat, and reduce your sugar intake without feeling as though you're on a diet. My program will help shift your thinking away from the negative mindset of "forbidden" and "bad" foods to a more positive attitude around the many "good" foods that you *can* eat. This shift will lead to a healthier relationship to food. You may be thinking that this is impossible, but trust me—by keeping it simple and keeping it real, you will achieve your goals. If you have always dieted and failed to reach your goal, then you have nothing to lose—try this new approach, built on the standards set by *Eating Well with Canada's Food Guide* and my nutritional adviser and certified dietician, Carole Dobson.

Anyone who knows me knows I am constantly drinking water. I keep a water bottle in my car and gym bag, a glass on my desk at the office, and a Brita water carafe in the fridge at home. At the end of the day, I've enjoyed at least eight 8-ounce (250 mL) glasses of water. Yup, I might visit the washroom more often, but you know, my complexion is fabulous, my digestion is great, and I always feel pleasantly satisfied. I know that I am always flushing toxins from my body too, and it shows in my physique. My point here is that I have consciously chosen to drink a lot of water. It is part of my personal sensible eating plan and complements my healthy choices of nutrient-rich whole foods and snacks.

What you decide to put into your body has everything to do with achieving and maintaining a healthy and ideal body weight. Eating for good health is not about caloric restriction—it is all about achieving balance in your eating. In fact, when you strike that balance, you will feel fully satisfied in your brain and your belly and end up eating fewer calories and less unhealthy food. You will achieve the right balance of essential nutrients—carbohydrates, proteins, and fats—and the essential vitamins and minerals, and even preserve your bone density and youthful appearance (skin, hair, nails, and teeth).

If weight loss is your goal, then you need to learn and understand that losing weight is a metabolic equation around the calories you spend versus save. If you want to guarantee your chances for permanent weight loss, then you need to think differently about this calorie equation. You need to consume fewer calories than your body can burn, for a deficit at the end of the day. You will, however, need to choose your calories wisely so that you can build and maintain your lean tissue or muscle. The Newbody exercises will help you build muscle tissue, but you have to eat sensibly and eat a reasonable amount of lean protein to protect your lean muscle tissue against loss. The more muscle you make, the higher your metabolism will be and the more calories your body will burn, even at rest.

NEWBODY TIP: Count on muscle to boost your daily calorie burn and you won't have to count calories to lose weight. Make sensible food choices and you will have more energy to move and exercise daily.

Calories in (from food) + calories out (from daily activity and exercise) + basal metabolic rate (the number of calories your body burns as energy to sustain life) = overall calorie deficit or gain.

You want to spend more than you save when it comes to energy and calories.

MANAGE YOUR ENERGY AND METABOLISM

The two most commonly expressed desires among women are "I want to lose weight" and "I wish I had more energy." By learning and understanding the basics of energy and metabolism, you'll learn how to boost both. This will help you achieve your Newbody goals, whether they are weight loss, energy gain, or both.

As Albert Einstein observed, "the significant problems we face cannot be solved at the same level of thinking we were at when we created them." To be successful at losing weight and changing your body shape to make it leaner, fitter, and more youthful, you can't do the same things that you've been doing or even think about diet and working out in the same way that you have in the past.

Basal metabolic rate (BMR) is an estimate of how many calories your body needs to maintain its current weight. It accounts for about 70 percent of your total caloric expenditure and represents the amount of calories a day your body burns, regardless of exercise. (Your body burns calories to maintain the basic functions of life, such as pumping blood, breathing, digestion, and tissue repair.) BMR is influenced by weight, height, gender, diet and exercise habits, body composition (ratio of lean, fat-free weight to fat weight), and environmental temperature. As you age, your BMR naturally slows down by about 10 percent a year after the age of 40. To get a general idea of your BMR, here is a formula to use (and to calculate your daily calorie needs, multiply your BMR by 1.2 [high PA] to 1.9 [low PA], depending on your physical activity level):

$$655 + (4.3 \times \text{weight in pounds}) + (4.7 \times \text{height in inches}) - (4.7 \times \text{age in years}) = \text{BMR}$$

The good news is that you can alter your basal metabolic rate by moving your body more, exercising consistently, and building and maintaining lean muscle tissue and strong heart and bones—essentially the goals of the Newbody program!

So let's get you started on a healthy eating plan. My Newbody Sensible Eating Plan is a blueprint for your short-term success and long-term health. Without having to count calories or deprive your body of the nutrients it needs, you'll be able to cut out 250 to 500 calories a day just by following the Five Ps Please program, which is the basis of my Newbody Sensible Eating Plan. This can add up to about 1 pound a week, since 1 pound of fat is equivalent to 3500 calories. As you feed your body with nutritious whole foods, you'll also be able to take control of your cravings and restore your hormonal balance. These improvements together will help fire up your metabolism and create a calorie deficit. To ensure that your goals are realistic and your nutritional needs are being met, I would encourage you to do a little homework and learn about nutrition, or speak with a dietician, especially if you have any health issues or concerns. Expert advice always pays off, which is another reason why I have worked with Carole Dobson, a certified and registered dietician, to develop my Newbody Sensible Eating Plan.

My approach to feeding your new body begins with making healthy choices and prioritizing your needs and your time so that you can take control of your cravings and restore energy and hormonal balance with food—and never count a calorie or be on a diet ever again. You will lose weight steadily and permanently at a rate of about 1 pound a week, but if you watch out for, and cut out, hidden calories—sugar syrups and cream in your coffee, salad dressings (particularly the "low" or "non-fat" types), added sugar in recipes, and condiments—you can further trim your caloric intake by up to 150 calories a serving—and double your weight loss. When you add the 30 minutes of daily exercises 6 days a week at 250 to 300 calories a session, you've also burned 1500 to 1800 calories a week from exercise alone, not to mention the increased metabolic demands down the road from building and maintaining muscle tissue. Add this deficit to your calorie-intake savings and double or triple your weight loss opportunity. There's no need to count them because they're gone!

THE FIVE Ps PLEASE PROGRAM

The five practical Ps for making healthy food choices are plan, portion, plate, prepare, put it to paper:

1. **PLAN**. You really are what you eat, and if you want to a build a new body, lose weight, and improve your health, you'll need to look closely at what you eat and follow a plan to make healthier choices. Without a plan, you will lose time, spend a lot more money and effort, and become frustrated with learning how to feed your new body a balanced, nutritious meal.

   The typical western diet we have grown up eating is often oversized and loaded with saturated and trans fats, refined sugars, artificial flavourings, preservatives (especially sodium), and processed to the point where there is virtually little to no nutrients left in it. In most cases, this is due to the fast-food phenomenon—and while many fast-food restaurants and food manufacturers are making healthy changes to their menus and products, there is still a long way to go.

   You'll need to plan not only *what* you eat but *when* you eat so that you're feeding your body nutritionally dense or "whole" foods in proper balance throughout each day. To do this, you need to eat less and more often—5 to 6 smaller meals each day. That means breakfast, lunch, and dinner along with 2 to 3 snacks. Each meal needs to include the following combination: a whole-grain/complex carbohydrate, vegetables and/or fruits, and a lean (high-quality) protein.

2. **PORTION**. You have to learn to control your portions to control your calories. This is a simple healthy eating strategy and there is no calorie counting required. If you don't have a plate to eat on (for example, if you're preparing lunch or snacks for on the road), you can get a good handle on controlling your portions by using your hand to size up amounts.

   - palm = lean protein (equivalent to 3 ounces, or 90 g)
   - fist = fruits and grains (equivalent to 1 cup, or 250 mL)
   - hand (open with fingers spread) = veggies (2 cups, or 500 mL)
   - thumb = fat (1 ounce, or 30 g)

Take a look at my plate as a guide to divide your plate the same way.

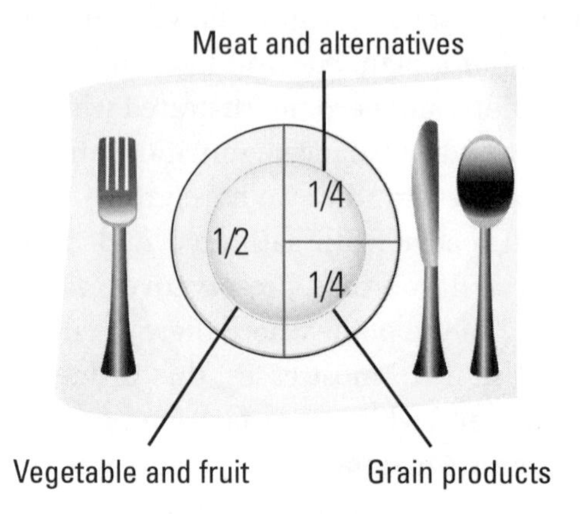

Each section represents one of the main food groups and its recommended portion size: fruits and vegetables take up one-half of the plate; whole grains and starches take up one-quarter of the plate; and lean protein takes up the remaining one-quarter. Each of these food groups plays an important role in managing your body's needs. Eating the proper balance of the essential nutrients (complex carbohydrates, healthy fats, and lean, high-quality protein) is significant in the weight loss equation (build and maintain muscle, lose fat), allows you to feel satisfied and full of energy, and is important for the health of your organs and the balance of your hormones.

3. **PLATE.** Size matters when it comes to controlling calories, cravings, hunger, and hormones. Simply downsizing your plate size (from a 12-inch plate to a 9-inch plate, or from a 10-inch plate to a 7-inch plate) and filling it using my portion size guide, you can retrain your brain to feel full. When the amount of food that you're eating looks big, it acts as a visual cue and tricks the brain into thinking that you're eating more. As a result, you feel satisfied rather than restricted (which is what you feel when you're on a diet). One reason diets don't work is that you're always focused on restricting yourself and you end up developing cravings that get out of control. Now it's time to take back control of your eating habits. Divide up your portion

sizes as you prepare your meals ahead of time and pro-actively prepare and put your leftovers away before you eat. When eating out, ask the server to divide up and prepare a doggie bag with half the entree, so that you can take it home with you for the next day. Or try doing what my husband and I often do at a restaurant, and order a salad each and one entree to split. This will help you take control of how much you eat at any one given time.

4. **PREPARE** to eat sensibly. It all starts with what you put in your shopping cart, allow in your kitchen pantry and refrigerator, put in your lunch bag, and have readily on hand for snacking. Preparation is essential to your success. Choose from healthy sources so that you're consuming whole foods in a rainbow of colours and rich in the essential nutrients that nourish your new body. Refer *to Eating Well with Canada's Food Guide* to learn how to build your own healthy meal. It doesn't have to be gourmet, just nutritionally balanced with respect to food groups—they need to be proportional in serving size to one another. Be sure to make a list before you go grocery shopping. Going shopping without one often leads to overspending on items you don't always need or already have at home. If nothing changes in your choices, nothing changes in your body. This may take a little time, but you won't regret it. You'll quickly see that you save time in the end. You'll most likely spend less time in drive-through lineups and eat more healthily in the progress. The extra time you save in looking for lunches and snacks you can spend on your Newbody workout!

5. **PUT IT TO PAPER**. Keep a daily food journal and record in your journal what you put into your mouth. This food journal will become your future meal planner, and it'll be especially handy on busy days when you don't have time to plan. Looking back at past daily logs and repeating what you did well is one of the most proven ways to take control of your eating. Keeping a food journal will also help you learn about your personal association with food and improve your willpower, lifestyle, habits, and results. There's more about writing down your goals and actions on paper in Chapter 1: The New and

Improved You, and I have created the Newbody Journal and the Newbody Eating Planner Sheet that will get you started and keep you on track. See the appendices (pages 210 and 212) for templates that you can cut out and copy.

NEWBODY TIP: Self-monitoring is key in managing your weight. Studies consistently demonstrate that self-monitoring your eating and exercise is critical in managing weight loss and maintaining weight loss long term. Most people will naturally underestimate their energy (food) intake by about 30 percent and overestimate their energy output (physical activity) by 50 percent. Consciously monitoring each and then writing down actual numbers on paper will give you an accurate picture and also help you see a pattern in your behaviour.

THE KISS OF GOOD HEALTH

This quick overview outlines the health benefits you can achieve just by making sensible and healthy eating choices. Always eat the healthier option, and eat for the new body that you want. Here's a "keep it simple, succeed (KISS)" checklist to make sensible eating easier.

NEWBODY TIP: Put this list on your refrigerator to help you measure a 1 portion serving:

Fruit

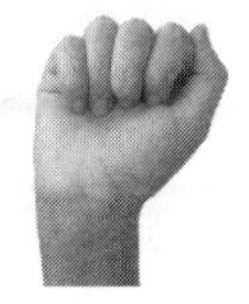

1 medium-size apple, banana, orange
1/2 cup (125 mL) cooked/canned fruit (unsweetened)
3/4 (175 mL) cup fruit juice

Vegetables

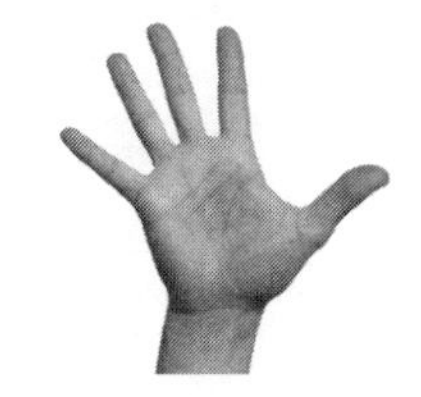

1–2 cups (250–500 mL) raw leafy greens
1/2 cup (125 mL) other vegetables cooked/canned
3/4 cup (175 mL) vegetable juice

Milk/Dairy:

1 cup (250 mL) milk or yogurt

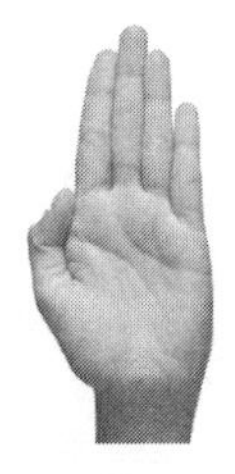

1 ounce (30 g) natural cheese

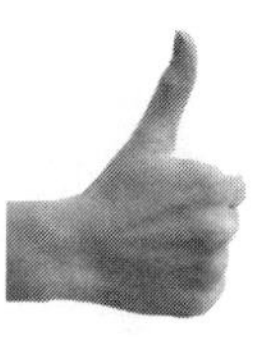

Meat/Poultry/Fish/Eggs/Nuts/Beans

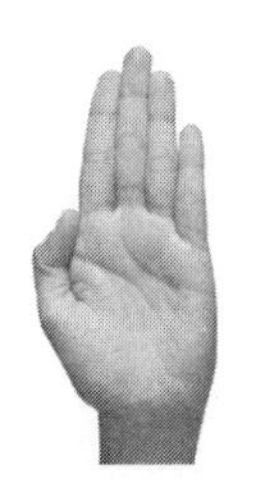

1/2 cup (125 mL) beans
2–3 ounces (60–90 g) cooked lean meat, poultry, fish
1 egg
1 ounce (30 g) prepared meats
1 tablespoon (15 mL) peanut/almond butter

Bread/Cereal/Rice/Pasta

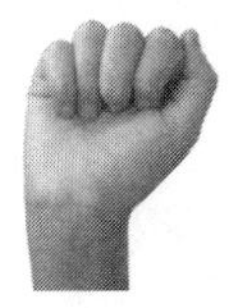

1 slice of whole-grain bread
1 6-inch pita wrap
1 cup (250 mL) cold cereal
1/2 cup (125 mL) cooked cereal/rice/pasta

Newbody Goal	Don't	Do
Balance blood sugar and hunger and energy level	Drink coffee and other caffeinated drinks excessively—reduce caffeine intake to less than 200 mg/day. (200 mg = 2 cups of coffee or 5 cans of caffeinated beverages)	Graze by eating smaller portions more frequently (5 to 6 mini-meals a day) that are balanced in nutrients (whole grains/starch, a vegetable/fruit, and source of protein); drink water and eat low-glycemic foods including apples, pears, berries, whole grains
Restore metabolism and reduce weight	Skip meals or diet (don't restrict your caloric intake to less than 1200 calories a day); go back for second helpings; snack within 2 hours of bedtime	Graze by eating smaller portions more frequently (5 to 6 mini-meals a day) that are balanced in nutrients (whole grains/starch, a vegetable/fruit, and source of protein); control portion and plate size; always eat breakfast; drink eight to ten 8-ounce (250 mL) glasses of water daily
Reduce/control food cravings	Eat for comfort, eat out of habit, or skip meals	Snack or graze every 3 to 5 hours to manage energy and blood sugar levels; achieve balanced nutrition at every meal
Reduce cortisol response/ maintain healthy hormonal levels	Consume more than 200 mg of caffeine or 1500 mg of sodium a day (200 mg of caffeine = 2 cups of coffee or 5 cans of caffeinated beverages; 1500 mg of sodium = 2/3 teaspoon. Basically, don't bring the salt shaker to the table); consume excess refined grains, simple (processed) carbohydrates, artificial sweeteners and preservatives, and artificial and trans fatty foods	Eat high-quality protein and consume high levels of antioxidants from citrus fruits and vegetables; use herbs instead of salt on foods
Feed your muscles and build new lean muscle	Skip out on protein in an attempt to cut calories; consume carbohydrates and fats for energy	Consume high-quality protein and healthy fats; eat a mixed-nutrient (carbohydrate with a protein) snack within 1 hour before and after exercising

Newbody Goal	Don't	Do
Build immunity and lower risk for illness and diseases (heart, stroke, cancer, diabetes)	Consume too much sugar	Get the daily recommended amount of vegetables, focusing on a wide variety of dark, orange, starchy, leguminous, and others; take a daily multivitamin and mineral supplement that includes antioxidants
Staying hydrated for toned skin and muscles, and energy	Consume caffeinated beverages	Drink eight to ten 8-ounce (250 mL) glasses of water; eat 5 to 10 servings of fruits and vegetables a day
Lower LDL ("bad" cholesterol)	Eat foods that contain a lot of fat or are high in saturated fats	Top up on your 5 to 10 servings of fruits and vegetables a day; eat low-fat dairy, lean protein, and whole grains
Build strong bones, healthy hair, and strong nails	Consume excess caffeine and sodium; smoke	Be sure to get 1000 to1200 mg of calcium and 200 to 400 IU of vitamin D (10 minutes of sun exposure) every day; eat foods containing healthy fats; consume at least 2 cups (500 mL) skim or 1% milk, or fortified soy beverage plus 1 more serving of dairy (milk, yogurt, or cheese) or alternative (calcium-fortified) beverages (soy, rice, orange juice); eat lean non-dairy protein (beans, canned salmon) and vegetables or fruit at every meal and snack
Improve your memory	Consume excess red wine, chocolate, and caffeinated beverages; skip meals	Eat small meals more frequently throughout the day; be sure to include protein and complex carbohydrates at each for better concentration and alertness
Improve your quality of sleep	Consume excess caffeinated or alcoholic beverages; eat big meals late in the day	Eat a complex carbohydrate snack (with protein and calcium) of less than 200 calories within 2 hours of bedtime

ONLINE NUTRITION TOOLS AND TIPS

There are many science-supported resources and nutritional plans available online that I refer to on a regular basis. These sites can be very helpful if you wish to learn more about sensible and balanced nutrition and even learn how to create your own healthy meal plan. Here's a selection:

- Health Canada's *Eating Well with Canada's Food Guide* at www.hc-sc.gc.ca
- Canadian Heart and Stroke Foundation at www.heartandstroke.ca
- Canadian Diabetes Association at www.diabetes.ca/about-diabetes/nutrition
- Canadian Dieticians' Association at www.dieticians.ca/eatwell

Eating Well with Canada's Food Guide is a population-based guide. This means that it is meant to cater to all Canadians. One of the wonderful new changes since the latest edition of the guide is that the "largest" food group is now fruits and vegetables. These foods provide you with the most nutrition, and the best part is that they have the fewest calories. The guide promotes "real" or "basic" foods. Most of the foods in your diet should be real or basic foods and not prepared, packaged foods. Following the guide ensures that you are meeting all your daily goals for micronutrients (vitamins and minerals) and macronutrients (carbohydrates, proteins, and fats). The guide recommends that you time your nutrient intake, eat 6 small meals each day or eat every 3 to 5 hours to help keep your blood sugars stable throughout the day. This is the most sensible way to control cravings, sustain your energy, manage your mood, and even balance your hormones.

STRIKING THE HORMONAL BALANCE

It is common for some women to turn to food for comfort, especially when stress levels rise. This isn't initially all bad because your favourite cup of java, peanut butter and jelly sandwich, cookies, and chocolate (in moderation) give your body what it needs at the time and this is one step toward managing stress. But doing that in a healthier way will better prepare you for combating stress while at the same time controlling cravings.

Unfortunately what tends to happen is that we let our comfort eating get out of control—and this leads to food cravings that begin that proverbial downhill slide that throws off our delicate hormonal balance. When hormones are out of whack, metabolism crashes along with energy, mood, and self-esteem. We gain weight and feel guilty and unhappy and that leads to more comfort eating—and the vicious circle continues to spin out of control.

On the inside, your adrenals (glandular organs that sit on top of your kidneys) produce three hormones: norepinephrine, epinephrine (also known as adrenalin), and cortisol. The norepinephrine and epinephrine cause several changes in your body that help you survive stressful situations, giving you a burst of energy for the "fight or flight" response. But insulin release is also halted so that you'll have lots of blood sugar available for energy. Your appetite takes a back seat as your heart rate and blood pressure rise and your body is on high alert. As soon as the stress has passed, cortisol takes over and tells the body to stop producing norephinephrine and epinephrine; your blood sugar drops off quickly soon after; and together, that kicks your appetite into high gear.

This short-term survival response mechanism is a good thing—however, too much of a good thing becomes a bad thing, as my mom would say. Unfortunately, this response mechanism occurs in response to almost all stressors—from skipping meals and dieting, feeling depressed, or feeling premenstrual to work deadlines and traffic jams or lineups that make you run late. When stress is always present (chronic), your body can't get rid of the excess cortisol and it builds up in the bloodstream along with sugar. The cortisol hangs around, wreaking major havoc on your body and your health—the worst of it is that it causes fat storage around the belly.

Food cravings for high-fat and processed carbohydrates (simple carbohydrates with loads of sugar) is your body's first response to stress, and when you give in to these cravings, your brain signals "victory" to your body, secreting rewarding chemicals that make you feel good. This sets up an addictive unconscious response with food—you feel stress, you eat, you feel better. This becomes part of your body's continual response to stress, which leads to chronically high levels of cortisol.

To create a new body and lose that stubborn, dangerous fat around your middle, you will need to retrain your body's response to stress so that you can keep your cortisol levels under control. You can do this by eating healthy foods and developing healthier responses to stress—the most important being to exercise. You must also, of course, exercise as well as eat sensibly if you have weight to lose. This excess weight is the dangerous kind that not only slows your metabolism by playing fast and loose with your hormones but also raises your risk for health problems including life-threatening diseases. By learning how to control your body and brain's stress response and creating new habits around cravings, you can take back control of your hormones and manage your metabolism better. If you've got extra pounds to lose, you will find weight loss so much easier when you combine your efforts with regular exercise. You'll manage your energy better, maintain a healthier digestion, regain your mental focus and clarity, and reduce the negative impact of stress on your body—both inside and out.

You know that your hormones are in balance when

- You have mental clarity and focus and experience positive feelings about yourself and the world.
- Your memory serves you well and you don't have headaches or migraines.
- Your skin is acne-free, vibrant, and hydrated.
- Your body weight and moods are stable.
- Your energy level and sex drive are stable and strong.
- You have healthy digestion.
- You are pain-free in your muscle and joints.
- You sleep soundly and wake up refreshed.
- You experience minimal to no premenstrual or premenopausal symptoms.

NEWBODY SNACKING STRATEGIES TO CONTROL CRAVINGS

- **SNACK, NIBBLE, AND GRAZE YOUR WAY THROUGH YOUR DAY**—to feed your body and maintain good energy, balanced blood sugar levels, and an active metabolism.

- **KEEP A FULL WATER BOTTLE ON HAND** in the car or at the desk and sip on that to curb your craving.

- **SNACK OR NIBBLE ON SOMETHING NUTRITIOUS** before you go to a staff or business meeting or a cocktail party and stand away from the food; take up conversation right away and you will be less apt to snack on the wrong types of food. Snack 1 to 2 hours before you exercise and within 1 hour after exercise.

- **PREPARE YOUR SNACKS** as you would your main meals for the day. This will make or break your control. If you become hungry or have cravings between meals, your chances of staying in control are far better if you can feed your craving with a snack that you planned and prepared beforehand. If you give in to the craving, it is more likely that you will throw in the towel and binge. The timing and type of snacks will help or hinder your new body success. Always include the proper balance of healthy complex carbohydrate and a source of protein in your snack to feed your brain, blood, and muscles the fuel they need.

- **WAIT BEFORE GIVING IN TO YOUR CRAVINGS.** Make yourself wait 15 to 20 minutes because the temptation to give in to cravings weakens and becomes less frequent when you outlast your feelings for a quick, gratifying release of pleasure: sugar. On the other hand, it is sometimes important to respond to your craving, as it is your body's way of correcting a deficiency—especially if you're exercising and depleting your body of glycogen (the storage form of carbohydrate in the muscle). It may be a minor deficiency, so it's better to meet that need than eat everything and anything else—and end up eating more—in the attempt to satisfy what your body really lacks.

- **COMMIT TO 15 TO 20 MINUTES OF LIGHT ACTIVITY FOLLOWING A BIGGER MEAL** (lunch or dinner) and perform light duties (go for a walk, do light office or household chores), water your plants, or practise your dance steps. This time will lower your chances of snacking later by greater than 50 percent.

- **BRUSH YOUR TEETH DIRECTLY AFTER A MEAL**—especially dinner, when late-night cravings tend to surface. Food is less appealing after the taste of toothpaste is in your mouth.

- **EAT EVERY 3 TO 5 HOURS** and curb mindless snacking by avoiding snacking while standing, talking on the phone, working on the computer, watching television, driving, or running errands. You will not have your mind on what or how much you're eating. This is a sure way to pile on the calories without realizing it.

- **AVOID LATE-NIGHT SNACKING** and eating just before bed, as this will disrupt your quality of sleep as well as lead to weight gain in the long term.

- **AVOID TALKING YOURSELF INTO CRAVINGS.** Learn how your brain thinks about food cravings and seek to understand your body better. Here's a perfect example: tell yourself (out loud), "I can't eat chocolate." Now what are you thinking about? That's right: chocolate, and now there's a good chance you'll be fixated on that until you get some. That is why diets fail and cravings prevail. Your brain focuses on what you can't have and it only thinks about wanting it. That being the reality, focus on what you can and want to eat versus what you can't eat. Make the choice *not* to go on a diet. Instead, go for sensible, balanced eating and include healthy, whole foods. Follow the Five Ps Please Program to control caloric intake, your hormones, and your metabolism. Don't count calories—count steps, for example, if you need something healthy to replace your old calorie-counting habits. Give yourself flexibility to allow yourself some treats while not giving in to your cravings. Plan for one treat a week and make it part of your plan—and don't feel guilty for enjoying it. If you have a bad day and fall off your plan, don't stress about it (this will make your cravings worse). Instead, move your body to move your mind away from the negative and make a fresh start tomorrow. Journal your feelings around food and exercise and refer back to learn what works, what doesn't, and what sticks for you with regard to food and your feelings around it.

- **MOVE YOUR BODY.** Physical activity is essential and guaranteed to control cravings as well as burn calories. It helps regulate blood-sugar levels and stimulate the brain's secretion of endorphins (those happy hormones that make you feel good). These brain chemicals improve mood, energy levels, and self-esteem, and these responses create a distraction for food. Your muscles divert blood away from your stomach and hunger dissipates. You will be more apt to make sensible decisions around food following exercise. Make sure, however, that you refuel with a healthy snack or meal within 1 hour of exercising to manage your metabolic needs.

- **MANAGE YOUR STRESS.** If your life is full of stress, it can and will be difficult to make sensible and healthy eating choices because food becomes a source of comfort. Many women respond to stress by under- or overeating, eating unhealthy food, consuming too many calories at one time, and abusing alcohol and other substances that cause negative hormonal responses that lead ultimately to weight gain, diabetes, heart disease, and stroke. Recognizing this negative and vicious cycle is the first step. Reprogram your mind and your body to stressors in your life by replacing negative habits with new, positive, and healthy actions.

Q&A *with* Mo

Q Do I need to eat protein bars, and do you have any suggestions about healthy ones and what to look for?

A I don't believe that you need to be eating protein bars to be healthy or to help you lose weight. But protein bars can make a great snack because they contain carbohydrates as well as protein, and as I mentioned before, having protein in a snack is essential for regulating blood sugars, preventing cravings, and keeping you feeling full and satisfied. If you choose to eat a protein bar, choose one that provides less than 200 calories, or only eat half of it if it has more. Avoid protein bars that have "coatings" on them (they look like chocolate bars with added protein). The more basic, the better (my favourite is the Elev8te Me bar).

Q I want to eat healthily but I feel I'm way too busy—how do you eat healthily with a hectic schedule?

A A little planning goes a long way! It has been proven that people who take a few minutes to plan their meals and snacks each week have much better success at eating more healthily and losing weight. Take 10 minutes with your husband or significant other—or even your kids—to plan lunches and dinner for at least 5 out of 7 days of the week. (Breakfast should consist of your favourite breakfast foods. If you don't eat breakfast, plan to start because that will set you up for eating more healthily all day.) Make sure that when you leave the house, you always carry a healthy snack containing protein. That way, if you're out for a long time or if you get hungry, you'll make a healthy choice. Put your plan to paper and you'll be more apt to stick with it. Make up your grocery shopping list after you've planned your meals and buy only what you need that week. Everyone has the same amount of time in a day—1440 minutes, to be exact. If you take a little time planning, you'll not only save calories, you'll save money and time in the end.

Q Do energy drinks really work? Should I use them to keep my energy levels up during my workout?

A Energy drinks are not sports drinks. They contain high sugar levels, and the fizz (carbonation) in energy drinks can make it hard to drink enough to stay well hydrated during a workout. The caffeine in energy drinks is usually more than double that in soft drinks. Caffeine will make you alert for a short time but tends to be followed by feelings of low energy. Too much caffeine can also get in the way of a good night's sleep, which is the real key to long-lasting energy that will get you through your day and your workout. Also, the effects of artificial ingredients mixed with caffeine are not well known so I would recommend you avoid energy drinks. The better choice is a sports drink, as they are designed for rapid hydration and refuelling during exercise. They are mostly water with some sugar, minerals (electrolytes), and flavour. They can help keep energy levels up when exercise is long and hard or when you sweat a lot. For shorter workouts, water is your best choice for hydration—and, of course, it contains zero calories. The best choice for keeping your energy up is having a healthy and nutritious snack containing high-quality protein 1 to 2 hours before exercise and within 1 hour after exercise. Here are my favourite healthy pre-workout snacks (be sure to drink one 8-ounce/250 mL glass of water with each snack):

- A small bowl (1/2 cup/125 mL) of whole-grain cereal or granola with 1/2 cup/125 mL low-fat yogurt and 1/2 cup (125 mL) of berries or half a sliced banana

- A protein smoothie made of 2 scoops of lean protein powder (or 1/2 cup/125 mL of skim milk or yogurt), 1/2 cup (125 mL) of berries, 1/2 cup (50 mL) orange or cranberry juice, and crushed ice, blended
- A half a bagel (multi-grain or whole wheat) with turkey, lettuce, 2 slices of tomato, and mustard
- 1–2 mini whole-wheat pitas with tuna, cheese, or peanut butter with banana, or sliced hardboiled egg
- A high-fibre cereal bar with a piece of cheese and a handful of raisins, or a small piece of fruit

Q If I exercise, does it matter what I eat?

A Yes, it does—and in some ways, it matters even more because your body will crave nutritious foods with protein (for muscle repair and growth), healthy complex carbohydrates (for energy and mental focus and clarity), healthy fats (for organ function and energy), and water (to rehydrate). Proper nutrition will help you build a leaner, stronger, and healthier body faster than exercise alone.

Appendices

APPENDIX 1

NEWBODY JOURNAL FOR THE WEEK OF: ______________________

MY GOAL IS: ______________________

Exercise Checklist (✓)							
	Monday	**Tuesday**	**Wednesday**	**Thursday**	**Friday**	**Saturday**	**Sunday**
Newbody 30-minute Workout							
2–15 minutes Extra Strength Training							
Additional Physical Activity (minutes)							
Total Physical Activity Time (minutes)							
Sensible Eating Checklist (✓)							
Breakfast							
Morning Snack							
Lunch							
Afternoon Snack							
Dinner							
Optional Evening Snack							

	Monday	Tuesday	Wednesday	Thursday	Friday	Saturday	Sunday
	Quick Nutritional Checklist (✓)						
4 Protein (meat/milk/ alt) Servings							
3–4 Fruit Servings							
4–6 Veggie Servings							
5–6 Grain Servings							
8 Glasses of Water (circle)	1 2 3 4 5 6 7 8	1 2 3 4 5 6 7 8	1 2 3 4 5 6 7 8	1 2 3 4 5 6 7 8	1 2 3 4 5 6 7 8	1 2 3 4 5 6 7 8	1 2 3 4 5 6 7 8
1 Glass of Alcohol/ Beer (or less)							
I Feel Success (Yes/No):							

One thing I am proud of this week:

APPENDIX 2

NEWBODY EATING PLANNER SHEET

Plan/Prepare each meal by selecting food and serving size from the list (in the left column) and placing it in each meal category below.

FOOD GROUP/PORTION SIZE/ FOOD ITEM	Plan/Prepare 5–6 smaller meals each day as per *Sensible Eating Plan*
Choose 2 Unsaturated Fats/Oils Thumb/2–3tsp Salad-type oil—1 tsp Soft margarine—1 tsp Canola/olive oil—1 tsp Peanut/almond/nut butter—1tsp	Breakfast—Choose 1 Protein and Grain, 1 Fruit and/or Vegetable serving and Water (1 glass)
Choose 4 Protein (lean meat/dairy/ alternative) Palm/3–4oz Lean meat Skinless poultry (turkey/chicken breast) Fish (tuna, salmon, white) Dairy 3/4–1 cup, 175–250mL Egg—1 Low fat cottage cheese, yogurt, skim or soya milk *Thumb/2–3oz* Cheddar, feta, goat cheese, mozzarella	Morning Snack—Choose 1 Grain, Fruit or Vegetable serving and Water (1–2 glasses)
Choose 3–4 Fruit Servings Fist/1 cup/250 mL Apple (med) Peach/Pear/Orange (med) Apricots (3 fresh) Avocado (1/2) Grapes (15–20) Banana (med) Kiwi (large) Grapefruit (1/2) Tomato (med) Fruit juice (125mL/1/2cup)	Lunch—Choose 1 Grain, Protein, 1 Fruit and 1–2 Vegetable servings and Water (1 glass)

Choose 4–6 Vegetables in Variety of Colors ***Open hand/1–2 cups/250–500mL*** Mixed vegetables—raw and cooked *Green:* Broccoli, spinach, romaine lettuce, mesclun mix, asparagus, peppers, beans *Orange:* Carrots, sweet potatoes, winter squash, pumpkin, yams, peppers *Yellow:* Beans, peppers *Red:* Beets, peppers	**Afternoon Snack**—Choose 1 Grain, Protein, 1 Fruit or Vegetable serving and Water (1–2 glasses)
Choose 5–6 Grains ***Fist/1 Cup/250mL*** Whole grain bread 1–2 slices High-fiber bran/oat muffin—1 small Whole-wheat bagel/English muffin/pita bread—1/2 Cooked whole-grain pasta/oatmeal cereal 3/4–1 cup Cooked brown/white/wild rice–1/2 cup Cold high-fiber cereal 3/4–1 cup Plain popcorn—2 cups	**Evening/Dinner Meal**—Choose 1 Grain, Protein, 2 Vegetable servings, 1/2 to 1 Fruit serving and Water (1 glass)
Choose 8 glasses of water ***1 cup/250mL***	**Evening Snack** (Optional)—Choose 1 Grain, 1/2 to 1 Fruit or Vegetable serving and Water (1 glass)

APPENDIX 3

GOODLIFE FITNESS® 1-WEEK GIFT MEMBERSHIP

GoodLife FITNESS® **FREE 7 DAY GIFT MEMBERSHIP**

$30 VALUE

Guest Name: ______________________

Guest Membership Card Start Date: ______________________

Guest Membership Card Expiry Date: ______________________

Membership Co-ordinator Name: ______________________

Lose Weight, Feel Great & Live Longer! 1-800-597-1FIT • goodlifefitness.com

*Must be 18 years and older. Other restrictions may apply, see club for details.

Acknowledgments

Newbody Workout for Women was written in recognition of all the Newbody instructors and thousands of Newbody participants with whom I have had the honour and privilege to teach, train, and work over the last 20 years.

To the 250-plus (and growing) instructors: it is because of your dedication to the Newbody program that it has become what it is today. Your passion for this unique total body fitness program has inspired thousands of participants to get healthier and fit! The stories shared by participants throughout the book are truly inspirational. Their success reminds me that fitness is not just about getting into better shape and losing weight; it's so much more than that. It is about building a lifestyle rich in health and vitality, inside and out.

Before writing this book, I contemplated for many months what I would write about. I asked myself what I could share with women that would help transform their mindset and approach to fitness. While more and more women are turning to fitness as a means to achieve their personal health goals, unfortunately a large majority of Canadian women still don't exercise regularly enough to achieve and maintain optimal health. Heart disease continues to rise and is the number-one killer in Canada. Young women and girls, some less than 10 years of age, often suffer potential life-threatening issues around body size and self-image. It is my hope that the Newbody workout, along with my sensible eating plan, will help mothers, daughters, sisters, and their girlfriends achieve health and fitness for life.

Newbody has allowed me to live my dream. It has enabled me to travel around the globe teaching people how to move their bodies with a joy for living and a zest for life.

Thanks to all those who have influenced my journey with Newbody, beginning with Lexie Williams (Australia), Patch, and all the instructors and members for their trust in me; to those who have provided me with the opportunity to connect with women through articles and interviews, such as Gilda Swartz and Ylva Van Buuren; to my mentors and coaches, who have guided and supported me in my journey; and to my husband, Ken, whom I love dearly. He was very likely the first man to participate in my Newbody class, more than 15 years ago. And the rest, as they say, is history.

Index